DOCTORS
of the OLD WEST

True Tales of the Old West

by

Charles L. Convis

Watercolor Cover by Mary Anne Convis

PIONEER PRESS, Inc., CARSON CITY, NEVADA

Copyright © 2005 by Charles L. Convis
All Rights Reserved
Manufactured in the United States of America

Library of Congress Catalog Card Number: 96-68502

ISBN 1-892156-19-9

CONTENTS

SKILLFUL SOLDIERS (Lewis and Clark)	2
PAVLOV'S PREDECESSOR (Dr. William Beaumont)	4
OPEN-AIR CLINIC (Marcus Whitman)	8
FIFTEEN WOUNDS BUT IMPROVING (Dr. John S. Griffin)	10
ELIMINATING COMPETITION (Dr. Edward Willis)	13
ROUND TRIP TO THE GOLDFIELDS (Dr. James L Tyson)	14
BUT OH, I HAVE SUFFERED (Dr. Ellis Reynolds Shipp)	18
HERO - INVENTOR - GERM FIGHTER (Dr. George Sternberg)	23
THE LITTLE DOCTOR (Dr. William W. Mayo)	28
DETERMINED TO BE A DOCTOR (Dr. Bethenia Owens)	34
USEFUL BONES IN NORTH DAKOTA (Dr. Henry Wheeler)	36
MY DEAR MOTHER (Dr. Holmes O. Paulding)	38
DOCTOR GRANDMA (Emma French)	42
FRONTIER NEUROSURGERY (Dr. George McCreery)	45
HOUSE CALLS IN A BIG HOUSE (Dr. Susan Picotte)	46
AGENCY DOCTOR (Dr. Thomas Bailey Marquis)	50
DOCTOR SOFIE (Dr. Sofie Herzog)	52
DOC SUSIE (Dr. Susan Anderson)	54
SWAT THE FLY (Dr. Samuel Crumbine)	56
BESSIE AND THE BRONCO (Dr. Bessie Lee)	57
ORDERING INFORMATION	62

ILLUSTRATIONS

DR. ELLIS REYNOLDS SHIPP	19
SIOUX CHIEF CUT NOSE	31
DR. HOLMES O. PAULDING	39
DR. SUSAN PICOTTE	47

SKILLFUL SOLDIERS

Neither President Thomas Jefferson nor his two captains considered a physician necessary for the Corps of Discovery. Meriwether Lewis's mother practiced herbal treatment in Virginia, and her son had a better background of medical knowledge than many physicians at the time. In addition, Jefferson arranged for Dr. Benjamin Rush, America's foremost physician, to instruct Lewis. The expedition's medical supplies included fifty dozen bilious pills, developed by Dr. Rush.

Only one man died on the 8000-mile, four-year expedition, Sergeant Charles Floyd. Very likely he had appendicitis. Since abdominal surgery was unknown at that time, a physician would have made no difference. Floyd's treatment, if any, was not described. The usual administration of calomel or bilious pills would have ruptured an acutely inflamed appendix.

Sacajawea, wife of the expedition's interpreter, benefitted from an excellent treatment which seemed to follow an incorrect diagnosis. The sixteen-year-old new mother, who joined the expedition in North Dakota, had a serious medical problem described in diary entries on June 10, 1805. Clark wrote: "Sacajawea, our Indian woman, is very sick. I bled her."

Clark did not describe her symptoms, but bled her again the next day. She complained all one night, and by the 15th she seemed dangerously ill. Clark "gave her the bark (Peruvian bark, a source of quinine) and applied it externally to her region which revived her very much."

But the next day they worried more, and Lewis took over the girl's care. He wrote: "I found that two doses of the bark and opium had produced an alteration in her pulse for the better; they were much fuller and regular. I caused her to drink the mineral water altogether."

The diary entries on the girl's treatment have been studied by Dr. Howard P. Holt of the Yakima Valley in Washington. He wrote; "(Sacajawea's) pulse had been barely perceptible, very quick, frequently irregular and attended with strong nervous symptoms of twitching of the fingers and leaders of the arms. She was complaining of lower abdominal pain. She began showing signs of improvement. Lewis made a diagnosis of 'an obstruction of the menses and consequence of taking cold.' He remained in camp to care for her."

Dr. Holt considered Lewis' treatment impressive. He said the girl had a fluid and electrolyte imbalance caused by vomiting and diarrhea, which was corrected by the mineral water. She got the right treatment for the wrong reason and she recovered. Fortunately she got sick at the portage at Great Falls where she was able to get the long rest she needed.

Another medical achievement for the expedition was the survival of

Sacajawea's baby who was only two months old when it started. The baby was sick on May 22, 1806 (returning from the Pacific). Lewis wrote: "Charbonneau's child is very ill. He is cutting teeth and for several days past he has had a violent lax, which being suddenly stopped he was attacked by a high fever, and his neck and throat were much swollen this evening. We gave him a dose of cream of tartar and flour of sulfur, and applied a poultice of boiled onions to his neck as warm as he could bear it." Dr. Eldon Chuinard, whose medical review of the expedition is accepted by scholars, said good doctoring, good mother's care, and good luck saved the baby.

The treatment with cream of tartar and sulfur continued until June 5, when Clark applied "a plaster of salve of rosin of the long leaf pine, beeswax, and bear oil which (cured) the inflammation entirely." Three days later the child was nearly well. Dr. Holt said the child must have had cellulitis of the neck which did not abscess and drain. The warm packs and his mother's care saved him.

Boils and dysentery plagued the expedition. They used herb compresses on the boils, occasionally draining one. Purging with calomel or Rush's pills was the standard treatment among physicians for dysentery.

When one man accidentally cut a large vein on his leg, Lewis applied a tourniquet with a cushion of wood below the wound. With the bleeding stopped, he closed the wound with ordinary sewing needles and thread. The man recovered completely.

Lewis was almost killed on August 11, 1806, when one of the hunters mistook him for an elk in dense brush and shot him in the thigh. He doesn't reveal the treatment, but almost a month passed before he could walk without pain.

Once, they found an Indian boy who had been abandoned in the cold. Ten days later, Lewis took off the toes on one of the boy's feet. Still later, he amputated the toes on the other foot. He must have used a carpenter's saw as they did not have a surgeon's saw.

Clark treated Indians with bad teeth and sore eyes. He developed a reputation among the Indians as a medicine man of strong power. He also helped a paralyzed chief walk with what appeared to be heat therapy and manipulation of his limbs.

Excellent medical care became an important part of one of the greatest exploring expeditions in world history.

Suggested reading: Howard P. Holt, M. D. *Saddle Bag Medicine* (1984.)

4
PAVLOV'S PREDECESSOR

William Beaumont, raised on a Connecticut farm for his first twenty-two years, left home in 1807 looking for excitement. He taught school for a time and then apprenticed himself to Dr. Benjamin Chandler, a leading physician in St. Albans, Vermont.

The apprentice ground powders, rolled pills, polished surgical instruments, and swept and dusted the office. When his master amputated an arm or leg, Beaumont kept the grisly trophy, carefully dissecting the nerves, blood vessels, and lymph vessels, and studying the bones and muscles in the evening by candlelight.

Four years later, his training finished, Beaumont joined the Army medical corps to serve in the War with England. He fought at Niagara and Plattsburgh, New York, and received a citation for bravery.

He practiced medicine in Plattsburgh and fell in love with Deborah Green. Bored with civilian practice, he rejoined the medical corps and was sent to Fort Mackinac in 1820. The fort, on an island where Lakes Huron and Michigan meet and near the strait into Lake Superior, guarded the gateway which thousands of voyageurs, mostly French Canadians, passed through to the western mountains.

A year later Beaumont married Deborah and brought her to the fort. A year after that, during a typical voyageur revelry on June 6, 1822, a shotgun roared and the medical officer had enough excitement to last the rest of his life. The charge of buckshot hit nineteen-year-old Alexis St. Martin in the stomach. He dropped immediately, and bystanders beat out the flames as his clothing ignited from the arm's length shot. The bystanders, who had often seen violent death, agreed that St. Martin could not survive.

Parts of the man's stomach and both lungs protruded from the gaping hole in his midsection. A soldier ran for Beaumont, who was shocked when he arrived to see a piece of lung as large as a turkey egg and a portion of the stomach as large as a fist. The load of shot had driven wadding, clothing fragments, and pieces of bone into the young man's body. Food oozed out of the stomach through an orifice as large as Beaumont's forefinger. He just cleaned the wound on the man who was apparently dying, and applied a superficial dressing.

But the young voyageur didn't die, and Beaumont resumed his care. He removed shot, wadding, and splintered bone. He worked the lungs and stomach back into place and applied pressure while St. Martin coughed. Then he re-dressed the wound.

"He can't live long," Beaumont said. "I'll check back in a couple hours."

But after the patient survived the initial shock, Beaumont brought his instruments and carefully removed more shot, clothing, and pieces of bone.

For several months the young man's tissues expelled more shot and bone chips. The doctor could not close the hole in the stomach, so he kept it covered with a linen compress to keep food from falling out. Eventually the tissue closed into a rude valve that kept the contents inside unless Beaumont pushed it open with his finger. Then he could drop in bits of food, pour in or extract liquid, and observe results.

When the Poor Fund of the town was depleted, Beaumont took his patient into his own home and began experiments. Only two days after the fateful shot, Deborah had given birth to a baby girl. Yet this young frontier wife of an unschooled man with a burning desire to learn about medicine gladly shared her home with the strange patient.

At that time the digestive process was a mystery. Some physiologists thought the stomach acted like a grinding mill, others a fermenting vat, others a stew pan. No one had even isolated gastric fluid for study.

After two years of experiments, St. Martin had recovered to where he could chop wood and do chores for the family. Beaumont faithfully reported all his experiments to the surgeon general of the Army. He learned that when his patient lay on the side opposite to the opening, Beaumont could look directly into the stomach and "almost see the process of digestion."

"I can pour in water with a funnel," he reported, "or put in food with a spoon, and draw them out again with a syphon. I have frequently suspended flesh, raw and wasted, and other substances into the perforation to ascertain the length of time required to digest each."

He used all the foods found in a frontier post for his studies — rice and barley; apples and oranges; meats, including lamb, turkey, salt pork, and roast beef; carrots, turnips, and potatoes; and bread, cake, and dumplings.

Finally Beaumont asked for a transfer to the East so he could get help from experienced scientists. But St. Martin was tired of being pushed and poked; tired of having things dropped into him and taken out for analysis. In 1825 Beaumont went on leave to Deborah's home in northern New York, and the experimental subject escaped to Canada.

St. Martin returned four years later, in 1829. By then Beaumont was stationed at Fort Crawford, Prairie du Chien, at the mouth of the Wisconsin River on the Mississippi. Although he had married and fathered two children, St. Martin couldn't keep up the strenuous life of a voyageur. He was willing to let Beaumont continue his studies in return for board and room for him and his family and a small income, which came out of Beaumont's pay. Beaumont could see that his condition had not changed — he still had the opening into his stomach, and now he was in good health.

For the next two years St. Martin feasted, fasted, stood up, laid down, rolled over, and let Beaumont drop food into him and take liquids out of him. The doctor watched the digestion process, recorded temperatures, timed events, tested stomach products, and wrote his reports. The uneducated man turned out to be a fine researcher as he continued making new discoveries.

Besides his duties as an experimental subject, St. Martin ran errands, chopped wood, fathered more children, and enjoyed the same health as an average man. But the doctor and his subject grew to hate each other.

St. Martin was tired of lying still in uncomfortable positions, and in fasting for hours only to have his hunger end, not by tasting pleasant food but by having it dropped directly into his stomach. As he came to understand his importance to Beaumont, he tired of being treated like a servant; he wanted to be a family friend.

Beaumont's reports increasingly referred to his subject's "villainous obstinacy and ugliness." Their growing hatred had one great side benefit for medicine. For the first time in history a researcher studied the relationship between emotion and digestion.

Fort Crawford was at least as wild as Fort Mackinac. Beaumont had no equipment but a thermometer, a few vials, and a sand bath (vessel to provide even heat to equipment used in chemical processes). Yet he made the most important contribution in understanding digestion before Pavlov, the Russian physiologist whose research on digestion fifty years later won the Nobel Prize. It is interesting that Pavlov, also an Army doctor, made openings into stomachs of animals so he could make the same observations that Beaumont made. It is also interesting that Pavlov's research on digestion led to his psychological studies for which he became world famous.

Beaumont had never studied chemistry, so he sought a year's leave to take St. Martin to Europe where the best chemists could be found. But Indian troubles around Prairie du Chien erupted into the Blackhawk War, and Beaumont treated wounded at the Battle of Bad Axe River. He returned to the fort, eager to go on to Europe, when a cholera outbreak further delayed him. By the time he got to Washington, his leave had been shortened to six months, so he had to complete his research in the United States.

St. Martin's wife, his staunchest ally in his battles with Beaumont, had moved to Canada with the children. Without her support against Beaumont's demands, the experimental subject began drinking heavily.

But the experiments continued, and Beaumont began reading physiology books. He had St. Martin's gastric juices analyzed by chemists in leading universities. They found that hydrochloric acid was an important ingredient, but they didn't know what else they contained. They urged Beaumont to send a specimen to the world's foremost chemist, Jöns Jacob Berzelius, in Sweden. Instead, Beaumont, trained only by experience, mixed hydrochloric acid with acetic acid and diluted the mixture with water until it tasted like gastric juice. Then he put chewed up beef in both gastric juice and in the chemical mixture and watched. The beef in the real juice dissolved; a jelly-like substance remained in the other vial. Obviously the real juice contained an unknown agent which completed the digestion. Three years later a German-trained medical researcher isolated the mysterious ingredient as pepsin.

Beaumont's descriptions of the stomach interior were the basis of all knowledge on that subject until the discovery of X-rays. Far ahead of his time, the doctor made discoveries about psychological aspects of digestion, including the effects of fatigue and emotion.

The doctor took his subject on tour, exhibiting him before groups of learned men. But the voyageur hated to stand exposed before strangers. Beaumont thought he was advancing knowledge by dragging his trembling subject before medical colleges, societies, and conventions. Eventually, however, St. Martin became so obviously miserable that Beaumont felt pity. He let him go home with the understanding that he would return for a tour of Europe.

St. Martin did not return. He wrote, "Me and my wife joins in love to you and your mistress and all the family. Hoping this may find you all in good health, I hope you won't be angry with me as I can do better at home."

So the strange partnership ended, but it had produced 238 published reports of experiments which made medical history. St. Martin certainly owed his life to Beaumont's surgery. Whether the benefits to medicine justified years of embarrassment and indignity to a Canadian voyageur, is a difficult question. The army doctor, isolated at a frontier fort, conscious of his own ignorance but blessed with a unique experimental subject, escaped the trap into which many experimenters fall. He sought the truth for its own sake, not to prove something he already thought to be true. He didn't know enough about digestion to have any preconceptions.

As a leading physician on the frontier, and now recognized as the first great American physiologist, Beaumont was soon earning between six and eight thousand dollars a year. He retired in 1839 after twenty-seven years in the army. He continued in private practice. In April, 1853, while calling on a patient in St. Louis, he slipped on ice-covered steps, struck his head, and died. He was a wealthy man.

St. Martin died twenty-eight years later, aged eighty. His family, having lived in poverty for many years, refused a large sum offered to place the world's most famous stomach in an army museum in Washington. To foil any attempt to disturb the body, they buried it eight feet deep in a secret, unmarked grave.

Suggested reading: James T. Flexner, *Doctors on Horseback* (New York: The Viking Press, 1937).

OPEN-AIR CLINIC

Marcus Whitman's father died in 1810, when Marcus was eight. The widow, with five children under twelve, asked relatives for help. Marcus left the family home to live with an uncle in Cummington, Massachusetts. Residing in the same small town was William Cullen Bryant, eight years older than Marcus and already a gifted poet. A year later, when he was seventeen, Bryant wrote *Thanatopsis,* one of the greatest poems in the English language.

The first time the word "Oregon" appeared in American literature was in these lines from Bryant's poem:

> Take the wings
> Of morning, pierce the Barcan wilderness,
> Or lose thyself in the continuous woods
> Where rolls the Oregon, and hears no sound,
> Save his own dashings . . .

We do not know how Bryant heard of the Oregon, the mysterious river of the West. Perhaps he had seen an English book in which Jonathan Carver wrote about Sioux Indians. Carver mentioned the "Origan," a river flowing to the Pacific Ocean. The name of the real river was soon changed to Columbia.

Whitman and Bryant, attending the same school, probably talked about the distant wilderness where the Oregon rolled silently to the sea. At any rate, when he was eighteen Marcus asked his family if they would help him become a Presbyterian missionary so he could serve in the Oregon country.

Presbyterian ordination required four years of college and three years of seminary. Marcus' mother and brothers could not afford such prolonged study. They persuaded Marcus to study medicine, instead, which required two years of apprenticeship to a doctor followed by one semester of formal study.

Marcus got his medical license and practiced in New York and Pennsylvania, but he never lost his desire to be a missionary. Finally, his dream came true. In 1835 the Presbyterian Board of Missions sent him west with Reverend Samuel Parker to look for a place where Marcus could serve as a medical missionary.

Whitman and Parker joined the caravan of the American Fur Company, traveling to its annual rendezvous, held, that year, on the Green River in present Wyoming. The rough mountain men resented the missionaries. They laughed at them for keeping the Sabbath. They tried to force liquor down their throats, and they threw rotten eggs at Marcus.

"I'm worried," Marcus told Parker. "We need these men to help get our missionaries to the West Coast."

"Let's hope and pray for the best."

In mid-June cholera struck. Marcus had had experience with the disease back in New York. He knew the importance of good sanitation and clean water.

Three men died, but Doctor Whitman saved all the others, including the leader, Lucien Fontenelle. From then on, the men followed the doctor's orders about camp sanitation, and he became the most respected man in the caravan.

They reached the rendezvous on August 12. Jim Bridger, the most famous of the trappers, asked Marcus if he could remove an arrowhead from his back.

"It's been paining for nigh on to three years now," Bridger said. "If you're a real doctor, mayhap you kin dig it out."

The next day, before hundreds of mountain men and about two thousand Indian observers, Doctor Whitman performed a difficult operation. A cartilaginous growth had "hooked" the three-inch, metal arrowhead into Bridger's spine. Working slowly and carefully, Whitman removed the object to the cheers of spectators.

Bridger, who had to drink his anesthetic, performed equally well. When Marcus expressed surprise that he found no infection in the wound, Bridger replied, "Meat jest don't spile in these hyar mountains."

For the rest of the rendezvous, Marcus doctored both Indians and whites. He won the respect and admiration of both races. Two of the trappers he met there, Bridger and Joe Meek, would later send their half-Indian daughters to be raised at the Whitman mission.

The respect won by Doctor Marcus Whitman became crucial to the successful introduction of missionaries into what is now Oregon and Washington. As settlers, miners, and businessmen followed, the country, originally occupied by the British, gradually became American.

If a teen-aged boy had not written a famous poem in Massachusetts, and if a doctor had not conducted a skillful, open-air, surgical clinic in the Rocky Mountains, Washington and Oregon would probably now be part of Canada.

Suggested reading: Clifford M. Drury, Marcus and Narcissa Whitman and the Opening of Old Oregon (Glendale: Arthur Clark Company, 1973).

FIFTEEN WOUNDS BUT IMPROVING

The battle of San Pascual on December 7 and 8, 1846, was the bloodiest ever fought on California soil. A few weeks afterward, the Californians surrendered and the land became part of the United States. The graphic account of an army doctor about the battle and his treatment of wounded resembles combat from the Middle Ages more than it does modern warfare.

Captain John S. Griffin, thirty, was orphaned in his native Virginia and raised by an uncle. He got his M. D. from the University of Pennsylvania at twenty-one. Three years later he joined the army as an assistant surgeon. After six years' service in the Seminole War in Florida and at Fort Gibson in present Oklahoma, he joined Stephen Watts Kearny's Army of the West to march to Santa Fe in the War Against Mexico.

New Mexico fell without a shot. Griffin accompanied two companies of the 1st Dragoons—about a hundred men—on to California where the story would be different.

After camping one day at Warner's Ranch in present San Diego County, the dragoons marched out on the morning of December 4. That evening they camped at the ranch of Edward Stokes, an Englishman who had settled there six years before. They laid over a day, then moved out on the morning of the sixth, guided by Stokes' foreman, Seignor Bill.

Marching in heavy rain, they met thirty-five sailors and Marines commanded by Marine Captain Archibald Gillespie, who had come up from San Diego. They camped in a live oak grove, and a four-man scouting party located the enemy about ten miles away.

The rain poured down during the night. The combined troops were out of their soggy beds and on the march at two a.m., hoping to surprise the Californians. Thirty men were left with the baggage and about a dozen assigned to Gillespie's four-pound gun. This left about ninety men and two howitzers to march on the enemy.

They crossed a mountain pass and saw enemy fires in the distance. They marched down the mountain and charged across an open valley. In the rainy, pre-dawn dimness, identification was difficult. A dragoon drew his saber and was about to cut a man down when Griffin yelled, "Stop, that's one of the Marines."

The Californians retreated a half-mile, halted, then rallied after the dragoons had fired their pistols (or had them misfire in the rain). Then the Californians charged "like devils with their lances."

The first casualty Griffin saw, Lieutenant Thomas Hammond, had been wounded with a lance thrust through the ribs. Some distance away,

Griffin yelled to Hammond to fall to the rear and he would treat him. General Kearny shouted that he also was wounded, but waved Griffin away, shouting, "Look after the other men first."

Griffin wrote, "the devils got around me and liked to have fixed my flint." Then Griffin found Captain Gillespie who was wounded directly over the heart. Another captain yelled at Griffin, and the doctor had his hands full. He ducked under one flashing lance and drew his pistol as another Californian charged. The pistol snapped on wet powder. He drew the other but forgot that he had fired it without time to reload. He threw the empty weapon at the charging lancer, who veered away.

In all, thirty-five of the fifty men who engaged the enemy in hand-to-hand combat were killed or wounded. The dragoons drove the enemy from the field and set up their camp. Griffin worked tirelessly the rest of the day treating wounded.

The battle resumed the next morning. The dragoons drove the Californians from the top of a hill and occupied it for the next night's camp.

The next day the Californians sent out a flag of truce accompanied by some tea and sugar and a change of clothing for Captain Gillespie. The clothing had been sent from San Diego with three men whom the Californians had captured. The dragoons exchanged one of their prisoners for one of these three.

On December 9 the dragoons were eating mule meat while the Californians paraded out of range. A wounded man died on the tenth. He had been lanced through the abdomen. That evening the Californians tried to stampede a herd of wild horses and mules through the dragoon camp, hoping they would force the dragoon horses away. The dragoons shot one of the charging mules and enjoyed eating him as he was a fat one.

About 2 a. m. the eleventh, eighty Marines and a hundred twenty sailors arrived from San Diego as welcome reinforcements. The next day all the troops reached San Diego, and the battle was over. Gillespie was later told by a Californian in the battle that they had seventy men, twenty-seven of whom were killed or wounded.

All of Griffin's wounded were doing well except one man, Streeter, who had eight wounds in the neck, five in the chest, and one in each hip, and another, Kennedy, who had five lance wounds in his head. Griffin feared that Kennedy's skull was fractured and his brain inflamed.

Kennedy died on December 19. Four puncture wounds had penetrated the brain. In the post-mortem autopsy, Griffin found the entire left side of the brain softened with purulent matter forming almost down to the ventricles. Streeter with his fifteen wounds was improving slowly but still suffering terribly. All the other cases were doing well.

Griffin sent word to Andres Pico, the Californian commander, that he was willing to treat his wounded. Pico replied that he had no wounded.

The recovering dragoons had plenty of beef and mutton but were down to four ounces of bread per day and no vegetables. Griffin feared dysentery with that diet. They had a grand review on December 22. It consisted of twenty dragoons on horses that Griffin said would have been wolf bait anywhere else in the country, plus eighty or a hundred Marines and forty volunteer riflemen. It was the most grotesque cavalry parade Griffin had ever seen. The Marines were not used to horses, and the animals with enough energy for a little kick would unseat the rider easily.

But Griffin wrote: "The Marines are as fine a body of infantry as could be raised in the United States. They are well drilled, active, healthy young men." He also said the sailors "had no superior as to fighting — they didn't know what back out meant."

A dragoon died of fever on Christmas day. It appeared to be sickness, not from wounds. Streeter, the man with fifteen wounds, still suffered terribly. He was improving although a bone was still exposed. Of the Americans killed at San Pascual, only two were victims of gunfire; the rest died from lance wounds, an average of three wounds each.

On December 29 Kearny led six hundred men—including crewmen and Marines from four naval vessels, dragoons, volunteers, and Californians who had surrendered and changed sides—out of San Diego toward enemy headquarters in Los Angeles. They stopped at San Pascual and learned that wolves had dug up one soldier and eaten part of his feet. It took eleven days to reach the San Gabriel River, about a hundred miles north. There they engaged Californians in a skirmish in which one man was killed and eight wounded, one seriously. In a fight the next day, five more men were wounded.

This was the last of the fighting, followed by several days of confusion between General John C. Fremont, marching from the northwest, and Commodore Robert Stockton, marching with Kearny, about who was to be military governor of California. Griffin did not think they could muster one half of the dragoons who had marched from Santa Fe to California.

Kearny's men returned to San Diego on January 23. Streeter, still discharging pieces of bone, survived but couldn't walk until May 10.

Griffin resigned his commission in 1854 to practice medicine in Los Angeles. His sister married Albert Sidney Johnston, famous general who fought under three flags — the Texas Army, the United States Army, and the Army of the Confederacy. Doctor John S. Griffin experienced violent combat just like his more famous brother-in-law.

Suggested reading: John S. Griffin, *A Doctor Comes to California* (San Francisco: California Historical Society, 1943).

ELIMINATING COMPETITION

When Doctor Edward Willis arrived in Old Dry Diggings (now Placerville) from England during the California Gold Rush, he thought he was the first doctor in the booming mining camp. He hung a blue sign on his tent with brightly-painted gold letters saying:

SURGERY
Dr. Edward Willis, M.C.R.S.
Surgery and physic in all branches.
Sets bones, draws teeth painlessly, bleeds. Advice gratis.

Willis soon learned that he had competition, an American named Hullings. A tall, heavy man, sporting a black coat and Mexican sash around his bright-green, velvet *calzoneras*, Hullings demanded to see the Englishman's diplomas and certificates. Hullings, himself, had claimed to be a man of learning and ability, but it is doubtful that he ever had any training.

Hullings, usually too drunk to take a pulse, certainly could not perform an operation. Most of the medical problems in the mines were emergency surgeries. Hullings was about as successful as friends and tent-mates of the injured (or wounded) miners.

When Willis presented his papers, Hullings grabbed them, tore them in two, and discharged a full stream of tobacco juice into their owner's surprised face.

Willis demanded an immediate duel to prove his honor. Hullings accepted. The wronged Englishman proved his mettle and demonstrated the manual skill of the best surgeons. They faced off, one shot rang out, and Hullings fell dead.

If the mining camp had been using such records, one could say that Willis' first professional act was signing the death certificate for his competition.

The miners recognized a gutsy man of skill, and Willis soon had a booming medical practice.

Suggested reading: George D. Lyman, "Scalpel under three flags in California," in *California Historical Society Quarterly, v 4* (1925).

ROUND TRIP TO THE GOLDFIELDS

Dr. James L. Tyson was one of fifty passengers on the schooner *Sovereign* that left Baltimore on January 16, 1849, bound for Chagres on their way to California goldfields. The passengers included one other doctor and a preacher. Tyson's diary provides a vivid eyewitness account of the travel and medical problems faced.

Passing Cape Hatteras, a crewman was washed overboard, his body not recovered. They sailed through the Caicos Islands and the Windward Passage between Cuba and Hispaniola. After passing Jamaica they crossed bows with a brig. Afraid it might be a pirate ship, the passengers put on their swords and pistols and strutted around, trying to look formidable, while someone fired a large blunderbuss. The brig put on more canvas and sped away, its crew apparently thinking they were evading pirates.

On their thirteenth day, after passing through shark-filled waters, they sighted the Isthmus of Darien (now Panama). That night they anchored at Chagres and left the vessel. They took a steamer up the Chagres River until it ran aground on January 31. They continued by canoes to Gorgona, thirty-five more miles upstream. One sick passenger asked Tyson to treat him. He complained of fever, cholera, and other dire diseases, but the treatment was not revealed. The temperature was over ninety degrees, and the passengers were glad to leave the alligator-filled river at Gorgona. Most slept there in tents, although some, including Tyson, stayed in an old shanty that passed for a hotel.

A committee of five, including Tyson, hired mules and rode on to engage ship passage to California. They found two ships at Panama, one British and one American. They engaged passage to San Francisco on the British bark. They took the whole ship, paying $200 each for 17 Cabin vacancies and $150 each for 49 steerage vacancies. They disposed of their surplus tickets among the 150 people already awaiting passage. Tyson got free passage when the British vice consul installed him as surgeon for the voyage. The preacher got the same privilege.

Tyson recommended that travelers across the isthmus drink as little water as possible, substituting claret or ale, but nothing stronger. "If brandy is used," he wrote, "the blood, already fired by the fierce rays of an equatorial sun, cannot long endure the accumulated heat, and fatal disease will almost necessarily be the result."

Two days later, the rest of the party reached Panama and an old fashioned Yankee hurrah, repeated nine times, sounded from the bark as it started the long voyage to San Francisco.

They headed southwest to catch the trade winds. After nine miles they stopped at an island to take on fresh water. There some passengers climbed a volcano and others killed a huge boa constrictor. One man, carrying a bare dagger at his waist, accidentally stabbed himself. Tyson stopped the bleeding and dressed the wound but noted that the man did not seem to recover from the shock.

Tyson also treated a man who fell headfirst through a hatch into the hold. He recognized the man as one who had been sick at Panama and had "uncleanly habits." At Tyson's recommendation, the captain returned the man to Panama. Stowaways discovered were caught and returned, except for one for whom the other passengers took up a collection to pay his passage.

On February 18, they met a bark from New Bedford, out seventeen months on a whaling voyage. The crew, eager for news, did not know who the president was. On the 23rd the man who had stabbed himself died and was buried at sea, and other such burials would follow. Shortly after, they met a Peruvian brig which had been becalmed for ten days. They wanted fresh water and medicines. The captain refused the water, but Tyson provided some medicine.

Sickness continued—once they had deaths in two successive days—and Tyson got the cabins and hold throughly cleaned and fumigated. On March 29 they were at Acapulco, where one of the crew deserted. Also at that place they took on eighteen more gold rush passengers who had come overland from Vera Cruz. Some had been waiting two months for passage.

Mexican authorities, some with relatives in the shipping business, threatened to prevent the new passengers from leaving. The passengers already on board offered to attack the town and spike the Mexican guns in the harbor. The presence of a British Man of War, whose officers said they would intervene if the British bark was fired upon, settled the international problem, and the new American passengers were allowed to board.

They left Acupulco on April 1. Shortly after, the other doctor in the group from Baltimore had a strange request for Tyson. He was a native of Florida, an intelligent, world traveled, older man who had practiced many years in Cuba. He said he was tired of living and wanted his money—a few hundred dollars—delivered to the governor of California to help endow a hospital. He asked Tyson to write his will and then give him a fatal dose of opium. Tyson tried in vain to cheer the man. Then he prepared the will and helped the man sign it. The old doctor soon breathed his last and was buried at sea. There is no indication of the use of opium.

As they neared the Gulf of California some passengers contracted colds. For the next two weeks they beat northward against violent winds and heavy seas. On May 11, hungry, shivering with cold, and wrapped in all the coats and blankets they could find, they had their first views of Alta

California. They were about even with San Luis Obispo.

On May 18, a beautiful morning, they lay becalmed off the entrance to San Francisco Bay. It took all day to work their way in to the Golden Gate. A brig that left Baltimore a few days before them to travel around Cape Horn, arrived the same day. Their bark anchored in the bay among a fleet of a hundred vessels.

San Francisco was a city of tents with a few frame buildings. Practically all the ships in the harbor had been deserted by their crews, anxious to hunt gold. A boat to take twelve men ashore cost twelve dollars. The newcomer's first interest was a meal of roast beef, bread, butter, and coffee. They pitched their tents in a sheltered place overlooking the bay. Their bark's entire crew deserted and visited them. The next night the bark's captain fell overboard and drowned.

San Francisco's May climate was miserable. Its hot morning sun gave way to cold winds with blowing dust, followed by heavy fogs. Tyson treated many men with respiratory ailments. He thought the place would never become a commercial center. Benecia or Sansalito (Sausalito) were much better. He was sure Sansalito was destined to become one of the great cities of the Pacific, if not the greatest.

Thirty-one of the Baltimore passengers bought passage on a launch to Sacramento. On their trip up the river they passed thousands of waterfowl, millions of mosquitos, many antelope, and one wolf. Sacramento was filled with Mexicans, Peruvians, Chilians, Sonorans, English, French, Dutch, Russians, Swedes, Kanakas, and Chinese, in addition to Yankees and native Californians. Gambling was rampant, and miners could lose a month's income on the turn of a card. But violence, bloodshed, and theft were rare. Tyson did treat a man for a dislocated jaw, suffered while drunk.

The party paid $700 for a ten-oxen team to haul their luggage 75 miles into the foothills. They knew they had brought too much with them. Tyson thought that one set of work clothing, one change of underwear, blankets, tents, and tools were sufficient. Pausing a few minutes at Sutter's Fort, a rude structure of mud, they continued up the American River. It took four days to reach the dry diggings. They found the miners from Oregon particularly hard on the Indians, resulting, Tyson thought, from their experience at home. Californians would hire Indians to work their claims, but the Oregonians would hunt them and kill them.

Unlike most doctors in the gold rush, Tyson did not try mining. He set up shop immediately and was busy from the start. The principal diseases were scurvy, rheumatism, dysentery, and fever. He never lost a patient to sickness. But after a few weeks in the dry diggings, Tyson and three others rode north to check out the Yuba River.

The heat and mosquitos were terrible, Tyson learned that two doctors "in full practice" had died from fever, and his small party returned to the dry diggings. There he heard from miners that they needed a tent-hospital higher in the Sierra Nevada Mountains. In early July, leading a party of six, Tyson hauled supplies to a point fifteen miles from the snow at a point between the headwaters of the American and Bear Rivers. Before the small hospital was finished, he had six patients, one an Oregonian hauled six miles on a litter from his camp. Others followed, and Tyson was again busy.

He stayed almost two months, but he found the practice monotonous. In one interesting interlude, he was furnished a steer and asked to open polls for the election of a delegate to a convention for organizing a territorial government. He sent out notices and butchered the steer, but no one came to vote. The beef spoiled and the area had no delegate.

By late August most of the miners had moved on to other areas, and Tyson decided to check out the Feather River, further north. He found that country "cheerless and desolate. All was parched, waste, and flat, with the sun glowing like a furnace." Tyson did meet a man from Baltimore, spent the night at his lodgings, and enjoyed the hospitality. Then Tyson returned to Sacramento where he fell ill with fever and bought passage to San Francisco. For five days he took nothing but water and medicine. He was treated by a doctor from Baltimore.

When he recovered, Tyson felt he had satisfied his curiosity about California, he feared a relapse of the fever if he returned to the mines, and he decided to return home. He boarded the steamer *Oregon* on September 30 and sailed the next day. John C. Fremont and a half dozen other passengers left the ship at Monterey to attend the convention for which Tyson had failed to garner a vote. The ship had other dignitaries, but Tyson was most interested in a wealthy Spanish widow. But she had eighteen children and was engaged to a youth of twenty-four. "So much for Spanish women!" Tyson wrote.

Again, Tyson was appointed ship's surgeon. Within a few days he had fifty-seven patients needing daily treatment. Most had been at the mines and suffered from "the complaints incident to the country." One patient died.

Again crossing the isthmus by canoe and steamer, Tyson boarded an American steamer at Chagres. While stopped at Port Royal, Jamaica, he bought a Marmoset, a rare monkey from South America. He reached New York on November 11, almost ten months after leaving Baltimore. Tyson had to leave the little animal on board for twenty-four hours, so he turned it over to a steamer employee. That night it froze to death.

Tyson, remembering the California heat, didn't mention the irony.

Suggested reading: James L. Tyson, *Diary of a Physician in California* (Oakland: Biobooks, 1955).

BUT OH, I HAVE SUFFERED

Ellis Reynolds, who moved from Iowa to Utah with her Mormon parents in 1852 when she was five, became one of Utah's first woman doctors. Acclaimed as Utah's outstanding woman for a one-hundred year period, she founded a school of obstetrics and nursing and shared speaking platforms with Susan B. Anthony, Elizabeth Stanton, Clara Barton, Harriet Beecher Stowe, and many women from foreign countries. The last sentence of her autobiography reveals much about this remarkable woman.

On May 5, 1866, nineteen-year-old Ellis married Milford Shipp, ten years older than she. He had a wife at the time who had just left him and had been divorced from an earlier wife. But Ellis was deeply in love and married her choice of suitors in spite of warnings from Brigham Young that she had not selected well. Ellis knew that Milford was "good and noble, that his principles were pure, and his integrity unsullied." She considered their "hearts united in an indissoluble tie that the vicissitudes of time or sorrow could not sever." She thought there was no greater bliss than having the power to bring comfort to the person one held most dear in life.

Milford, Junior, (called Bard) was born the next February, the first of Ellis' ten children. Now she prayed to be a perfect mother as she had been praying to be a perfect wife.

The next winter the family moved to Fillmore, over a hundred miles away, where Milford opened a new dry goods store. Ellis had her sister, Anna, come to stay with her, as Milford traveled often.

In late February 1868, Milford announced that he had accepted the mandates of the Celestial Law of Marriage and would bring home another wife, Ellis' sister, Maggie. Ellis firmly believed plural marriage was a divine command from God, but this enormous and early test of faith shocked her. Second child William Austin was born a few weeks later on April 11.

That summer the family moved back to Salt Lake City, and, in December while Milford was away on business, the new baby died. In her despair, Ellis set out on a plan for self improvement. She rose every day at four for three hours of prayer and the study of books on health and nursing.

In May 1869, five days after Ellis gave birth to Richard, Milford left for mission duty in England, taking Maggie with him. Still bed-ridden from childbirth, Ellis rejoiced that her husband, a skilled preacher, would bring the message of salvation to many souls in far-off lands. Ellis took in a boarder to help with expenses and began teaching school.

In June 1871, Ellis wrote that she had just enjoyed a ten minute rest after completing her morning's work. It was the longest rest she had enjoyed for several weeks. She wondered how she had lived for two years without

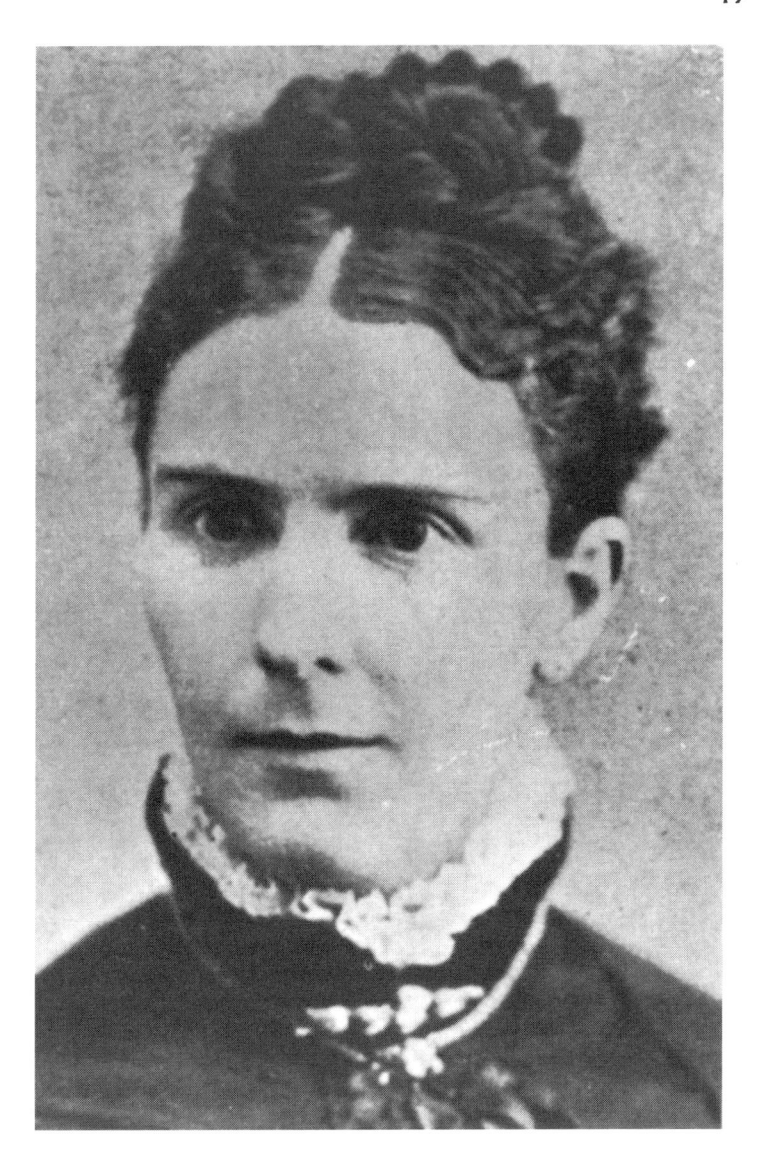

DR. ELLIS REYNOLDS SHIPP

Utah State Historical Society

Milford. She hoped her faithfulness would prove herself worthy of the full and perfect love of her husband.

The next month Milford returned from his mission. She met him in Ogden, and on their way home he talked to her about the principle of polygamy. Three months later he married Lizzie Hilstead. Ellis wrote that she tried to keep the spirit of God burning in her heart.

On the last day of 1871 Elliis wrote that she had complained too often. She prayed that she could use the next year to become a more true and faithful wife and a more kind and considerate mother. She still rose at four to study health and nursing. She still sewed six hours a day, making clothing for Milford's store. Milford had set out a course so that each of his wives could reach "the pinnacle of preeminence in his affection and esteem," but Ellis still felt discouraged. She tried with all her power and energy to follow in an undeviating line his instructions, but she wrote that clouds looked dark and her heart felt like it would break. "But thank Heaven there is one source of consolation — *Prayer.*"

A few days later, two days before her twenty-fifth birthday and in spite of her resolution to be cheerful and uncomplaining, Ellis spoke to Milford about the hardship of life. She thought many of the wives' trials were unnecessary when by a word or an encouraging look he could have made them happy. She even accused him of being partial among the wives.

Milford took a paper from his pocket and told her he had been writing some lines to present to her on her birthday. "These will show how wrong you are," he said, as he began reading.

His writing was elegant — full of pathos and feeling, Ellis wrote. It spoke of her patience and refusal to complain. She was the sunshine that drove his sorrows away. Oh, if she had only waited longer, the words would have been a priceless boon to her heart. She reached forth her hand, although aware that she didn't fully deserve the compliments. But he crushed the paper as if by the act he would obliterate every word, as if to free himself from any delusions he had about her uncomplaining nobleness. It was the most severe and cutting reproof Ellis had ever received. She felt as crushed as the paper.

The next April, Anna was born. Ellis was very weak for three weeks. The home had other children and babies, but Ellis doesn't say which were Maggie's and which Lizzie's. The three wives took six-week turns at being governor of the home.

Milford married wife number four, Mary, in February 1873. Ellis and Maggie made the wedding cake. On that day Ellis wrote that they were all so happy because their husband was so kind and generous, so noble, chaste and pure, and by his advice, counsels, and exemplary course leads his family in the path of truth and righteousness.

In May 1873, Milford went on a two-month mission to Arizona. He took wives Maggie and Mary with him. He also took six-year-old Bard. As parting gifts Maggie left Ellis a brooch, and Mary left Lizzie a beautiful box.

Two months after the family was reunited in Utah, Ellis' baby Anna died after a seven-week illness. Ellis knew that if she were true and faithful the baby would be restored to her in the angelic loveliness of Heaven but she still missed the prattling cherub who brought such joy to her often sad and weary heart.

Ellis was depressed and ill for four months after Anna's death. Then, in January 1874, nearing her twenty-seventh birthday, she resumed her heavy study schedule and started wondering if she had a mighty mission of her own to perform. Milford was away, and she longed for him. She knew his best wishes and prayers were with her and would ever be if she followed the wise and noble course he had so often advised. Again Ellis was up at four every day, but now, in addition to health and nursing, she studied grammar, rhetoric, and history.

In June, Maggie moved away, apparently returning to the home of their stepmother. Ellis never said why. Burt was born in September.

Ellis mentioned Milford many times in 1875 — his blessing the new baby, advising Ellis to stick to intellectual pursuits, confirming his oldest son as a member of the church, buying a farm where, with the help of his wives and children, he raised thousands of tomato plants and acres of corn — but she did not speak of him as a husband.

In November 1875, Ellis left her family to study medicine in Philadelphia. Milford wrote comforting, encouraging, and inspiring letters, and she thanked her Heavenly Father for such a husband. She was determined to succeed not only for her darling children but also for her dear husband.

Ellis thought she would dread instruction in dissection, but she found that every vein, muscle, tendon, nerve, and bone bore the impress of divine intelligence. She said, "Man is the greatest work of God." Still unable to sleep after four, she would go to the dissecting room as soon as it was light enough to see.

Ellis delighted in letters from Mary and Lizzie, as well as from her real sister, Maggie. By February 1876, she was getting *"glorious* letters from my dear husband." She had never heard such words of love and devotion from him before. She added, "Perhaps if I had heard them frequently, they would not seem so precious to me now." Ellis considered Milford "the ideal of perfect manhood, a Saint of God."

Milford came to visit in June 1876. Ellis was not in good health, and the college sent her home to recuperate. Embracing her children after the eight-month separation gave her one of the happiest moments of her life.

Pregnant, she returned to the medical college in September.

She was almost out of money when Lizzie sent some. Ellis wrote: "How pure and heavenly is the relationship of sisters in the holy order of Polygamy." But still exhausted and depressed, Ellis revealed her pregnancy to some classmates. "You don't need to go through with this," they said. "We could help you, you know."

Ellis' despair gave way to fury. "I came here to save life, not destroy it," she said. She spent all that night on her knees, praying for strength.

Milford sent his blessing for her confinement. She had a girl, Olea, on May 25. Two weeks passed before she could go up and down stairs. She felt blessed and grateful for Milford's letters. Lizzie had just had a girl baby about one month before. At this time Ellis was working hard on her thesis, *The Function of Generation.*

Still running short of money, Ellis was down to six cents when her sister Maggie sent ten dollars. Ellis tried to make money sewing, and she had an appointment in a hospital where she studied obstetrics and diseases of children. During one particularly instructive week she had three obstetric cases and helped in an operation for cancer, besides numerous other cases.

In March 1878, Ellis received her degree from the Woman's Medical College of Pennsylvania. Her trip home in a second class emigrant train with a new degree and a ten-month-old teething baby was a toilsome one. She began her practice immediately, a practice which lasted fifty years. She specialized in obstetrics and the care of women and children. She delivered over six thousand babies.

Ellis had four more children. Two girls, Ellis and Nellie, both survived their mother. Neither of the two boys, Ambrose and Paul, lived to be a year old. Bard became a doctor, Richard a lawyer, and the three girls, Olea, Ellis, and Nellie, all graduated from college.

The story of this distinguished woman is made up of three parts: her autobiography to age nineteen, her diary from ages twenty-four to thirty-one, and a reflective look back when she was eighty-three. At the end of her story she mentioned the doctrine of Plural Marriage. "I cannot say that I rejoiced," she wrote, "neither did I rebel, because of my implicit faith in the Gospel of Jesus Christ, which had been so thoroughly impressed upon my mind and soul." She said there still remained among the wives a most sacred bond of fellowship, a beautiful loving interest, and sweet affection one for another, that is most truly akin to the divine."

The last sentence in her book reads: But Oh, I have suffered, and pray it has never been in vain.

Suggested reading: Ellis Reynolds Shipp, *While Others Slept* (Salt Lake City: Bookcraft, 1985).

HERO — INVENTOR — GERM FIGHTER

Hartwick Seminary near Cooperstown, New York, the alma mater of George Sternberg, was the first Lutheran institution of higher learning in America, and it stressed the importance of high moral conduct. The seminary must have thought Sternberg met those standards when it selected him to give the principal address at its hundredth birthday celebration.

When Sternberg graduated from Columbia Medical School in 1860, he just wanted to be a country doctor and he started practice in New Jersey. A year later he joined the Union Army as an assistant surgeon. His behavior in the first Battle of Bull Run in Virginia in July, 1861, heralded a lifetime of bravery and devotion to his patients.

While Sternberg was treating wounded soldiers in facilities set up in a church, Confederates advanced, and the Union forces fled in a rout. The doctor refused to leave his men, and the Confederates captured him. Then he proposed a bargain: if the Confederates would allow him to continue his treatment, he would not try to escape for at least five days. The Confederates agreed, and Sternberg treated wounded from both sides. A little more than a week later, after his patients had stabilized, he escaped.

At the battles of Gaines Mill and Malvern Hill in spring 1862, his coolness in performing amputations under heavy fire while bayonets clashed nearby and lead flew overhead earned his reputation as a doctor with nerves of steel. He received brevets to captain and to major for heroism in the Civil War.

Sternberg was then taken from the battlefield and made executive medical officer of a 2200-bed hospital in Rhode Island. Now he had to fight another battle. Hospital gangrene, an infectious scourge of the Civil War, swept through the hospital, attacking both recovering soldiers and the fatally wounded. No one knew how it was transmitted. When standard treatment failed, Sternberg ordered his staff to use new, clean bandages on all wounds. Before then, doctors often used the same bandage on successive patients. He also set up quarantine wards and ordered all bodily discharges burned or buried. The entire hospital was scrubbed down, disinfected, and whitewashed, and patients received daily baths.

Some doctors laughed at the new methods, calling them Sternberg's housecleaning. But the gangrene epidemic was stopped. Sternberg had met his first epidemic and won.

Sternberg was surgeon-in-charge of a large, general hospital in Cleveland at war's end. The scientifically-minded captain liked army discipline, so he stayed in. By then he was also in love. Maria Russell from

Cooperstown was frail and unhealthy, but beautiful. They married in her home town in October, 1865.

After a short honeymoon, Maria and George moved to his new post, Jefferson Barracks on the Mississippi River at St. Louis. But their bliss ended the next April when Sternberg was transferred to Fort Harker, a frontier fort in Kansas. Maria's health was too fragile for such a place, so she went to live with her parents.

The fort, located on the Smoky Hill River, guarded the Santa Fe Trail. In the heart of hostile Indian country, it teemed with railroad workers, teamsters, buffalo hunters, friendly Indians, and immigrants. Sternberg treated all, many without pay.

By spring 1867, the railroad had reached the fort, and living conditions improved. A lonely year ended with Maria's arrival to join her husband. The fort became a beehive of activity as George Custer and the 7th Cavalry arrived to prepare for a summer campaign against Indians. Other troops passed through the fort to occupy newer forts further west, and battles flared all along the Smoky Hill. But life for the reunited couple held joy and excitement.

Then, on June 28 at 4:00 a. m. an ashen-faced acting assistant surgeon woke Sternberg from his sleep. A civilian working as the post butcher had been found in a dugout next to filthy slaughter pens. The man had collapsed from severe stomach cramps and said he'd had diarrhea for two days. His stomach and bowels had discharged a foul liquid.

Both doctors recognized the classic symptoms of cholera, a disease that had spread across the west the year before, killing 2,400 people. A soldier with similar symptoms already lay in the post hospital. Fearing an epidemic, Sternberg quarantined the butcher and the soldier. Before daylight, a teamster and a mother with her child were brought in with similar symptoms. By that evening all but the teamster had perished.

A gruesome silence settled over the fort as new victims, both soldiers and civilians, succumbed to the disease. Sternberg remembered his efforts to control gangrene in the Civil War. He had special tents set up for the sick in a quarantined area away from the hospital. Transient troops were moved away and kept by themselves. Soldiers who had been sleeping in two and four-man tents were put in single tents or in open-air lean-tos.

Each army company received a large tent to house men with symptoms of diarrhea. Soldiers policed the entire post, cleaning and disinfecting all latrines and sinks. All slop and garbage holes were cleaned and covered. Pine tar burned day and night. The dead were buried immediately.

Still the cholera raged. Sternberg and his two assistants worked around the clock without relief. On July 14, staggering with fatigue, he was summoned to his quarters. Cholera had struck his beautiful Maria. He worked over her frantically, but her health was too frail. Within twelve hours, his bride of less than two years—one of them spent apart—lay dead.

Sternberg had no time to mourn. Too many people lay suffering and dying. Doubling his efforts, he warned about drinking the river water. By now, civilian patients were crowding into the hospital, putting more strain on Sternberg and his overworked staff. Desperate, he asked the War Department for more help. A few days later, five doctors hurried into the fort. When they saw Sternberg, reeling from physical and emotional exhaustion, they ordered him to bed.

Thanks to the new doctors and faithfully following Sternberg's methods, the epidemic was short-lived, ending on August 1. But the cherished wife of a brave doctor was gone.

Just four days after Maria died, another officer, equally worried about his beautiful wife, rode into Fort Harker on a frantic dash from the west and boarded a train to Fort Riley where he found his wife well. But George Custer was court martialed for abandoning his command at Fort Wallace to see about his wife. The army found him guilty and suspended him from duty for a year.

With the epidemic conquered, Sternberg took leave and spent a few months with his family. In December, 1867, he was assigned as post surgeon at Fort Riley. This permanent cavalry post was the outfitting center for troops and supplies moving west. Here, Sternberg saw his first Indian fighting with Ben Grierson's storied 10th Cavalry and then rode as medical officer with Alfred Sully's expedition into Arkansas and Indian Territory to stop the illegal sale of whiskey to Indians. He served as medical officer on Phil Sheridan's winter campaign against Cheyennes, Arapahoes, Kiowas, and Comanches in Indian Territory in 1868-1869.

Between the campaigns Sternberg visited Indianapolis, where he met and courted a small, attractive woman, Martha Pattison. Sparkling with energy, she had a logical mind, and her interest in science delighted Sternberg. They married in September, 1869, and returned to Fort Riley.

The newlyweds were assigned to a large, old, run-down residence called the "Sutler's old house." Martha wondered why an officer of her husband's rank had been assigned to such undesirable quarters. Then she learned that he had traded to get the quarters because they provided him room to set up a private laboratory.

Sternberg spent almost all his free time searching for the secrets of infectious disease. He spent all his spare money on laboratory equipment and supplies. Soon his discoveries received acclaim from doctors in both medical and bacteriological fields.

Keeping weather records had long been part of Army doctors' duties.

Sternberg enjoyed the work and noted the effect of quick weather changes on the sick, particularly when prairie winds suddenly dropped the temperature. Realizing the benefits of stable environments, he tried building or smothering fires in patients' rooms as the temperature rose and fell. But the response was too slow; he needed some kind of heat regulation that acted quicker as temperatures changed. In the 1869-1870 winter he built a device known as Sternberg's Electromagnetic Regulator which combined a mercury thermometer, a magnet, and an electric circuit-breaker. He obtained a patent for the device, which now we call a thermostat.

Offers to buy the patent arrived, and Sternberg accepted one for $5000. He was on his way to Washington to transfer the patent and accept the money when another buyer showed up at Martha's door with an offer of $10,000. He pleaded with her to send a rider to overtake her husband. She said it would do no good, but he insisted. The rider caught up with Sternberg, who agreed with Martha that they were morally obligated to go through with the offer they had already accepted.

For the next six years Sternberg had assignments in New York, Massachusetts, Louisiana, and Florida. He battled one yellow fever epidemic after another, caught the disease himself, and nearly died from it. He weighed less than a hundred pounds when he recovered.

In 1876 he was transferred to Fort Walla Walla, Washington. Now a major with the title of surgeon, he hoped this fort would be a more permanent assignment. But the Nez Perce under Thunder Rolling from the Water up over the Land (the army called him Joseph) objected to loss of their lands, and the killing of a white, who had earlier killed an Indian, fanned a tense situation into war.

Sternberg marched to White Bird Canyon after the terrible defeat there and helped bury the army dead. Still not completely recovered from the yellow fever, he wrote Martha that he "was feeling quite well and stronger than when I started."

On July 11, 1877, the troops caught up with the Nez Perce at the Clearwater River, where Joseph decided to make a stand. The battle almost ended in an army disaster as great as the one at White Bird Canyon. While moving wounded from the battlefield during the night, Sternberg found one who had lost too much blood to be moved. He would have to operate right there to stop the bleeding. Indian sharpshooters on watch were so close the soldiers heard them talking. Sternberg had two men hold up blankets while he lit a candle and started to work. After a shot through the blanket, he blew out the candle and finished suturing the blood vessel by feel. He said nothing about the rescue—the man survived—and no officer saw it, so there was no recognition of his heroism until thirteen years later when the witnesses began to talk about it. Then the incident was added to his service record.

Later that night, wounded men pleaded for water, and Sternberg collected canteens and got volunteers to follow him to a nearby spring, right under the Indians' guns. For this he received a brevet to Lieutenant Colonel.

The Nez Perce finally broke off the fight and fled. General Oliver O. Howard ordered Sternberg to take the twenty-seven wounded to Grangeville, about twenty miles away. All he had were three broken-down wagons and some worn-out mules. Then he remembered the Cheyennes he had fought in Kansas. They had used travois to move people and property. He went to the deserted Nez Perce camp and recovered enough tipi poles to make travois on which he transported most of the patients.

Sternberg became so exhausted from loss of sleep that Captain Henry Winters of the escort assigned his orderly to ride beside the doctor and prop him up in the saddle. A temporary hospital in a community building served most of the patients but some needed better care, so Sternberg again moved the wounded in his little hospital train on to Fort Lapwai. The second night out on that ride, one man with a leg wound began bleeding heavily. Sternberg was practically out of medicines and drugs, but he knew the man could not survive without surgery. Without an assistant, and by candle light, he amputated the man's leg. The soldier survived.

While Sternberg was stationed at Fort Mason in San Francisco—a beautiful post, Martha said, for its view of the bay—he became the first American to demonstrate the tuberculosis bacillus. It was also discovered the same year by Robert Koch in Germany.

Sternberg's work in infectious diseases allowed him to work with such eminent doctors as Louis Pasteur, Koch, and Walter Reed. In 1881—at the same time as Pasteur—he announced the discovery of the pneumonia bacterium. He was the first United States doctor to discover the parasite that causes malaria and the bacillus of typhoid fever.

In 1893 Sternberg became surgeon general of the army. In that office he created the Army Medical School, the Army Nurse Corps, and the Army Dental Corps. He continued private bacteriological research after he retired in 1902.

Sternberg's heart had been damaged many years before when he almost died from typhoid, but he never let it reduce his effort. He died of heart failure in 1915, aged seventy-seven. The soft-spoken, white-haired old soldier had given the care of the sick everything he could. Recognized as the Father of American Bacteriology, he certainly lived up to the high standards of his alma mater, the academy where both his father and his maternal grandfather had taught.

Suggested reading: John M. Gibson, *Soldier in White* (Durham: Duke University Press, 1958).

THE LITTLE DOCTOR

A little man, five feet, four inches tall and slight in build, William Worrall Mayo was born in England in 1819. His father, a skilled joiner in a family of Flemish Protestants, died when William was seven. His mother came from a prominent family of Huguenots, French Protestants who had also fled to England for religious freedom. She saw that William got a good education. He studied medicine in England and Scotland, but came to the United States in 1845, before he got his license.

William found work in the Bellevue Hospital in New York City, and in 1848 drifted on west to Lafayette, Indiana. The next year he entered Indiana Medical College in LaPorte.

Medical education in the United States at that time was largely an apprentice system. A student would team up with a doctor to keep the office clean, care for the horses, mix his powders and salves, and watch him examine and treat patients. Two short sessions in a medical school were required for graduation, but graduation wasn't required to enter practice. Anyone could call himself a doctor.

One problem facing the schools was the obtaining of cadavers to use in their lectures. Indiana Medical College had an excellent reputation and drew students from all over the United States, but it got its cadavers like they all did — a few donated; many recovered in late night forays by students into graveyards, searching for fresh graves.

One unusual item of equipment at the college was a microscope, imported from England at great expense. Twenty years would pass before either Harvard Medical School or Johns Hopkins would have a microscope.

William got his degree in February, 1850. He returned to Lafayette and got his first job in a drug store, seeing customers who needed medical advice. He replaced a doctor who quit to follow the gold rush to California.

In February, 1851, Dr. Mayo married Louise Wright, a New Yorker of Scotch-English parentage. She had gone alone by canal barge and prairie schooner to visit relatives in Michigan when she was eighteen, and she met William when he was in medical school. She had little formal schooling, but read avidly and impressed all with her intelligence.

The next May, Mayo formed a partnership with the doctor with whom he had apprenticed earlier. Malaria was the worst of many sicknesses in the Middle West. The humid Wabash Valley was one of the worst areas for the dreaded disease. The connection between the disease and mosquitos had not yet been discovered. Dr. Mayo, himself, caught malaria.

But the many diseases in the area did little to increase business for doctors. Most persons relied on bleeding themselves or administering emetics, cathartics, and home-concocted remedies. Diseases had not been sufficiently differentiated for precision in diagnosis. Doctors relied on such terms as lung disease, liver complaint, inflamation of the bowels, and galloping consumption.

Surgery, also, had advanced little. Doctors were usually called only as a last resort. The public had little faith in them.

The Mayos' first child died at six weeks, a not unusual event at the time. Louise opened a millinery shop to supplement her husband's income. Louise soon outhustled her competitors and moved into a larger shop. When daughter Gertrude was born in 1853, Louise took on a partner so she could be spared for the domestic duties at home.

That fall, Dr. Mayo's partner joined the faculty of the University of Missouri Medical School in St. Louis. Dr. Mayo went with him as his assistant. The next spring Mayo had earned another M. D. But he and Louise had both come down with cholera, and he was tired of the malaria in the middle west. In summer 1854, he traveled further west looking for a land without chills and fever. He found it in Minnesota, and that fall he moved his wife and daughter to St. Paul. Louise opened a new millinery shop and immediately prospered.

With Louise supporting the family, Dr. Mayo explored Minnesota Territory. He spent all of the 1855 summer at Lake Superior. His employment varied from taking census to inspecting copper claims. He enjoyed canoeing in the northern lake country. He interrupted his explorations long enough to accompany Louise to New York and help her buy inventory for her store.

In fall 1855, Mayo explored southwest on the Minnesota River. He took over an abandoned farm across the river from Le Sueur. Louise sold her shop and joined him. He resumed medical practice, carrying his bag along narrow Indian trails to call on patients. At night, he carried a whale-oil lantern. Sometimes he rode a horse, but there were no trails for a carriage. Like most doctors, he had little income. He supplemented his practice with farming, treating animals, and running a ferry. A second daughter was born in summer 1856, shortly after they moved to the farm. A third daughter, born in spring 1859, lived only a year.

Life became hard for Louise Mayo after she gave up her shop in St. Paul and moved to the farm. She had to bake, cure meat and dry vegetables, can for winter storage, spin, weave, knit, mold candles, and make soap from lye leached from ashes with lard added. One day as she was cooking soap, she had a severe bleeding from the lungs. After she recovered she spent as much time outside as possible, and she became a good amateur botanist and astronomer.

Louise had to be brave with her husband gone so much to call on patients. The woods were full of wolves, wildcats, and bears. She never knew when she would see an Indian at the door to beg or at a window, his nose pressed to the pane to see what was inside. She caught trachoma and was almost blind for several years. Looking back later, she always described the Minnesota River Valley as "a hard country."

By 1859, Dr. Mayo had had enough of farm life. After severe flooding, he moved across the river to Le Sueur and built a small cottage in town. His first patient came while he shingled the roof. The farmer had a sick horse and wondered if he'd come.

"Sure will. I'll look at a horse or any other damn thing you got."

Le Sueur already had a doctor, Otis Ayer, a dour man about Mayo's age. When Mayo made the professional courtesy call, Ayer pointed out that the town wasn't big enough for two doctors.

"Why, Doctor," Mayo replied with an innocent look, "were you thinking of leaving?"

Mayo still had to supplement his income, and he worked on a steamboat on the Minnesota River the next spring and summer. He loved the rough life on the river. He met James J. Hill that summer. The future railroad builder was clerking on another boat. Mayo also published a newspaper, not as financially successful as steamboating.

In June, 1861, the Mayo's first son, William James, was born. By then the nation was at war, and the governor of the nation's youngest state (Minnesota was admitted in 1858) offered a thousand soldiers for defense of the Union. But the next summer the outbreak of the Sioux took the minds of Minnesota Valley residents off the war so far away. They had their own war to fight.

While Mayo rode home after treating a patient, three Sioux Indians accosted him at a shallow ford and demanded his horse. He recognized one as Chief Cut Nose.

"Get away, you drunken fools," Mayo shouted. Cut Nose grabbed the horse's bridle, and Mayo lashed him with his riding whip. "Take that you thieving rascal." Mayo escaped his three attackers and galloped home.

The outbreak began after a hard winter when hungry Indians gathered for the annuity payments promised them. Agent Joseph Galbraith had the food, but the cash hadn't arrived yet. He said checking the rolls twice for two distributions was too much trouble, and he turned the Indians away.

After listening to their hungry children cry for food with the government warehouse full, the Indians asked for another meeting on August 15 with the agent and some traders. Galbraith asked the traders if they would let the food go on credit until the money arrived.

One trader, Andrew Myrick, speaking for the others said, "As far as

SIOUX CHIEF CUT NOSE

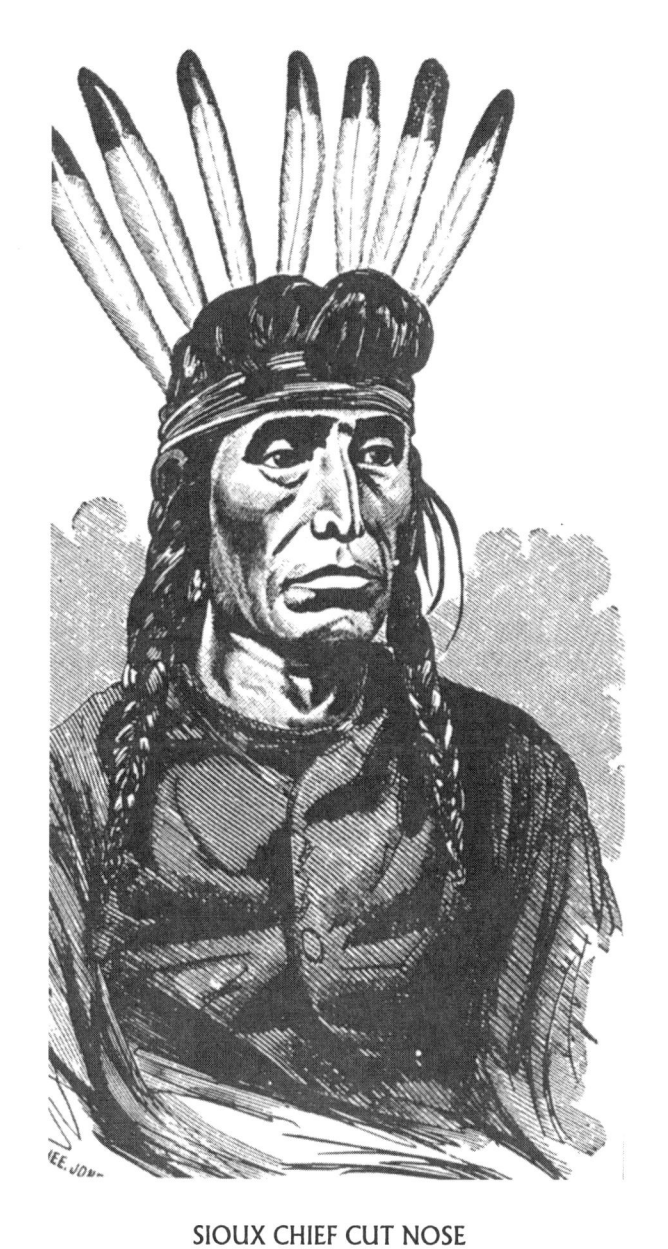

Leader in 1862 Outbreak in Minnesota

we're concerned, if they are hungry let them eat grass."

Two days later, four Indians killed five whites on a lonely farm. The next day a large band of warriors attacked the agency, killed all the men they could find and looted the stores. Myrick's dead mouth was stuffed full of the grass that he had insolently told the Indians to eat. Other Indians—seven thousand in all—ravished the Minnesota Valley, killing men, capturing women and children, gorging themselves with food, and burning barns and haystacks.

After a Paul Revere ride down the valley, a hundred twenty-five men organized to go upstream and fight. Dr. Ayer and another doctor carried medical supplies. Dr. Mayo marched with the riflemen and fought in one skirmish in which the Indians were beaten back after they killed thirteen defenders and wounded forty more. When they set up a hospital in New Ulm to treat the wounded, he joined the other doctors.

While he was amputating a leg, Dr. Mayo saw two men sneaking away from the battle. He ran out the door, brandished his bloody knife and ordered the men to get back to their posts. They did.

After the Indians withdrew, the whites moved back downstream to Mankato. There, those who could travel moved on toward St. Peter, but Mayo and another doctor stayed another week to treat the men who could not travel farther. Years later a man from Montana said that Dr. Mayo had saved his life when he was eleven.

"They took me to the hospital behind the lines," he said, "where a kindly little old man dressed my wounds and praised me for my courage. He was the Old Doctor Mayo. Everybody on the frontier called him the 'Little Doctor.'"

Meanwhile, Louise Mayo, alone with her three children, gathered the women of Le Sueur about her and told them to put on mens' clothing. They armed themselves with hoes, broom handles, and anything that looked like a gun, and tied on knives, spoons and anything shiny that would look like a bayonet. At intervals the women marched up and down the streets of Le Sueur, as though a defense force from Fort Snelling had arrived. The town was not attacked.

Louise took eleven families of refugees in to her house and barn. In one day she and little Gertrude baked an entire barrel of flour into bread for them. When she saw an injured man she would ask, "Who dressed your wounds." If he answered, "The little doctor," she knew her husband was still alive. He returned two weeks after leaving with the volunteers.

After a trial before a military commission, three hundred and seven warriors were sentenced to death. President Lincoln postponed the execution, and Minnesota citizens threatened to lynch the prisoners if they were pardoned. Lincoln pardoned all but thirty-nine. The evidence showed that they had committed rape and wanton murder. He ordered them hanged.

The execution of thirty-eight Sioux (one had died a natural death) at Mankato on December 26, 1862, was the largest execution in our nation's history. The bodies were taken down, dumped into wagons, and hauled to a hole dug in a sand bar in the Minnesota River. Half-bloods were buried in one corner so they could be disinterred by friends and family. The rest were buried in one pile.

Many doctors had witnessed the hanging and recognized a wonderful opportunity to obtain cadavers for medical schools and skeletons for explaining bones to patients in private offices. Dr. Mayo got the body of Cut Nose, the bloodthirsty warrior he had once bested in the struggle over Mayo's horse. Cut Nose had been a ringleader in the outbreak. Mayo dissected the body, cleaned it, articulated the bones, and used it in his medical practice.

In 1863 Mayo became examining surgeon for the enrolment (draft) board for the southern half of Minnesota, with an office in Rochester. Two years later he moved his family there. Their second son, Charles, was born in July, 1865, and the father then opened his medical office.

Like all American doctors at that time, Mayo was a general practitioner, but he liked surgery best. In 1869 he studied surgery at Bellevue Hospital in New York, where he had worked forty years before.

He was elected state president of the medical society in 1872. Many of southern Minnesota's doctors were sending their surgery cases to the Little Doctor, recognized as one of the best in the state. Louise, self-educated with his books and journals, had become one of his best assistants.

Will and Charlie, Mayo's sons, were well educated. They went to public and private schools. Their mother taught them botany and astronomy. They learned about bones from the skeleton of Cut Nose. Their father also taught them physics and chemistry, subjects he had personally learned from John Dalton, England's eminent scientist who first discovered the atomic nature of matter. The boys also helped their father in an apprenticeship of many years.

Will graduated from the University of Michigan Medical School and Charlie from Chicago Medical College (later called Northwestern University Medical School). By 1889 all three Mayos were on the medical staff of St. Mary's Hospital, whose name was later changed to the Mayo Clinic. The little doctor had come a long way in American medicine, and patients from over the world still come to the Mecca for medicine which he and his sons started in Rochester, Minnesota.

Suggested reading: Helen Clapesattle, *The Doctors Mayo* (Minneapolis: University of Minnesota Press, 1941).

DETERMINED TO BE A DOCTOR

Bethenia Owens was three when her parents emigrated from Missouri to Oregon in 1843. She grew up as the family nurse. With a new baby arriving every two years, she often had a two-year-old in her arms and a four-year-old clinging to her skirts.

Small, slight of build, and a tomboy, she had great will power and endurance. At twelve she bet her older brother that she could carry four, fifty-pound sacks of flour. He helped her take on the load, and she walked off with it to win the bet.

Bethenia married Legrand Hill at fourteen and moved into a one room, unchinked log cabin with neither floor nor chimney. Her furniture consisted of a bed of one leg with the rails fastened into the walls, a shelf for a table, and three shelves for a cupboard. Her husband had a horse and saddle, a gun, and less than twenty dollars; she thought it an excellent start in life. Her "soul overflowed with love and hope," and she sang "dear old home-songs from morning to night."

Hill was a good hunter, and they always had plenty of game to eat. But he did little else. At sixteen Bethenia had a baby boy, George, but they lost their farm, moving in first with his relatives, then with hers. After four years of marriage, she divorced Hill. Bethenia found herself at eighteen, broken in spirit and health, back in her father's house in Roseburg, from which she had left with a happy heart and such bright hopes for the future.

The young woman, barely able to read and write, decided to return to school. Her older brothers and sisters took care of George while she attended school with the younger ones. Determined to earn her own way, she took whatever work she could find.

Soon she was teaching school at ten dollars a month. Three of her sixteen students were more advanced than she, but she took the books home and night and got help from a brother-in-law to stay ahead of her class.

That fall she entered another school and suffered humiliation when placed in the primary class in arithmetic. She had to recite with eight-year-old children. She soon advanced to the highest class.

Bethenia became a milliner and dressmaker. She worked a while with the best milliner in San Francisco and then returned to Roseburg, Oregon, with the latest fashions and became the best milliner there. She made enough money to send George to the University of California in 1870.

She still had a fondness for nursing, and she borrowed medical books from a doctor friend. Then she decided to go east and study medicine, herself. Her family felt disgraced at her decision and her friends sneered. They all told her that she made far more money as a milliner than she could ever expect as a doctor.

But Bethenia went anyway, enrolling at the Eclectic School of Medicine in Philadelphia. She hired a private tutor and got her degree. She opened an office in Portland to give electrical and medical baths. Her practice flourished; she put George through medical school at Willamette University, and helped a sister attend Mills College.

But Bethenia was still not satisfied. She wanted to treat herself to a full medical course in the "old school" and tour Europe. Her family and friends still objected, saying she would be rich at what she was already doing.

Armed with letters from senators, governors, professors, and doctors, she sought admission to the nation's most prestigious medical school. It had never admitted a woman, and she was turned down. But with the help of the country's most famous surgeon, she gained admission to the University of Michigan medical school. Averaging sixteen hours a day in lectures and study, she graduated in two years, missing only one lecture during that time.

After clinical work in Chicago, she returned to the University of Michigan as a resident physician. Her son, Doctor George Hill, joined her there for post graduate work, after which they toured Europe together.

Then Bethenia returned to Oregon, proud that she was a regular, university-educated doctor and no longer just a "Bath Doctor."

After three of the most happy and prosperous years of her life, during which she felt married to her profession, she re-met Colonel John Adair, whose father had been a friend of her father. She remembered him as a handsome boy with beautiful curly hair. They soon married in the First Congregational Church of Portland.

At the age of forty-seven Bethenia gave birth to a baby girl. Her joy turned to despair three days later when the baby died.

Colonel Adair was reclaiming tide land along the Pacific and building a farm. Living there with him, Bethenia practiced in a very remote part of Oregon. For eleven years she rode horseback to call on patients, except when the trails were impassable for a horse and she walked.

In 1900, when she was sixty, Bethenia returned to Chicago to earn a post graduate degree. This time, she found it difficult to attend lectures and clinics from nine until six, with more studies in the evening.

Five years later, she retired from medical practice. She took up temperance work with the WCTU, and campaigned for more exercise, shorter skirts, and against sidesaddle horseback riding for women. She died in 1926, aged eighty-six.

Suggested reading: Cathy Luchetti, *Women of the West* (St. George: Antelope Island Press, 1982).

USEFUL BONES IN NORTH DAKOTA

The James Brothers and the Younger gang rode into Northfield, Minnesota, on September 7, 1876, to make a spectacular bank robbery. They didn't know they would also contribute to the education of two University of Michigan medical students and to the office equipment of one of them for almost fifty years.

Henry Wheeler and Clarence Persons, seniors at the university, were visiting their freshman friend, Charlie Dampier, whose father owned the Dampier Hotel, when the eight-man gang rode into town. The gang, which included Clell Miller and Bill Chadwell, had been robbing banks and trains for over four years. The Youngers asked Chadwell, a Minnesota native, to scout out the First National Bank, across the street from the Dampier Hotel.

The robbers looked forward to this prize. The bank, one of the richest in the Middle West, was owned by two prominent Union Officers from the Civil War. Southern sympathizers in the gang hated them. The robbers probably thought Northfield resembled other towns they had raided. But its citizenry, valuing law and thrift highly, would fiercely protect their town and their savings in the bank.

At two p.m. Jesse James, Bob Younger and Charlie Pitts dismounted and entered the bank. Cole Younger and Clell Miller waited outside, holding the horses. Frank James, Jim Younger, and Bill Chadwell guarded the exit from the town, ready to protect the others as they fled with the money.

A hardware merchant, seeing the strange horses outside the bank, walked over to investigate. Clell Miller grabbed his arm and said, "Keep your mouth shut."

The merchant broke loose and ran down the street, shouting, "Get your guns, boys. They're robbing the bank."

Miller and Cole Younger mounted their horses, and the three guarding the streets joined them. They rode up and down, telling the citizens to mind their own business. The technique that worked so well with Missouri's citizens, gun shy from Civil War desperadoes, didn't fly in Minnesota. Dozens of men, young and old, grabbed weapons and took up positions to fight.

Chadwell was killed by a resident, and Miller by the visiting student, Henry Wheeler, shooting a borrowed army carbine from a second floor window in his friend's hotel. Wheeler also wounded Bob Younger. Some unarmed residents threw rocks at the robbers as they rode away. Besides the two killed, four were wounded. Only Jesse and Frank James escaped unscathed. A sheriff's posse killed one more the next day and captured the three Youngers, all of whom got life sentences. Two citizens of the town were killed.

Wheeler and Persons had been talking about the scarcity of cadavers at their medical school. When the shooting ended, more corpses lay on the ground and in the bank than the University of Michigan was likely to see in a year.

"Nobody's going to care about these two outlaws," Wheeler said. "Let's take them with us to Ann Arbor."

So the three students buried the outlaws in shallow graves. When Wheeler and Persons went back to school, they slipped out one night, dug up the bodies, nailed each one inside a salted barrel, and hired a nervous wagon driver to haul the barrels, marked "paint," to the railroad station.

About a month later, the Ann Arbor *Courier* ran a story about the two medical students who had the pleasure of carving up two genuine robbers. But the publicity went too far. Miller's father in Missouri showed up and demanded his son's remains. Too much dissection had made it impossible to tell one body from the other. So Wheeler and Persons gave Mr. Miller a bag of bones and said it was his son.

When they graduated in the spring, the young doctors discussed who should get the other set of bones.

"You shot him, he's yours," Persons said.

So they assembled the bones, shellacked them, and Wheeler took them to Northfield, where he opened his new medical office.

Two years later Wheeler entered the College of Physicians and Surgeons in New York City, graduating in 1880. He then opened an office in Grand Forks, North Dakota, and practiced there until he retired in 1923. He was the seventh president of the North Dakota Medical Association.

Wheeler used the skeleton often in his medical practice. It helped explain anatomy and surgical procedures to patients. It remained in his office after retirement as an interesting conversational piece until the building burned in 1925.

Later called the Holstein Capital of America, and now home to St. Olaf's College and Carleton College, Northfield, for seven minutes in a violent afternoon in 1876, contributed a useful artifact to the office of a North Dakota doctor. He didn't know whether it was Miller or Chadwell, but he got good use from it.

Suggested reading: William Bender, Jr., "You Shot Him — He's Yours," in *A Treasury of True* (New York: A. S. Barnes and Company, 1956).

MY DEAR MOTHER

Dr. Holmes O. Paulding, twenty-three-year-old assistant surgeon in the regular army, was the only doctor in Gibbon's command as it marched down the Yellowstone in 1876 to meet Terry's command, marching up from Fort Lincoln. Gibbon had six companies of the 7th Infantry, and four companies of the 2nd Cavalry. Terry's command was larger, containing five companies of the 6th Infantry and the entire 7th Cavalry. It was the first time in its history that all twelve companies of the 7th Cavalry had marched together. Their march ended in disaster, and many details of the tragedy came from the letters of Doctor Paulding to his mother.

Paulding was annoyed with Gibbon's reluctance to engage Indians. When they located a large camp, he wrote: "Our genial commanding officer did not deem it advisable to attack it, a chance any other commander would give any price for."

After the Indians challenged them for ten days, Gibbon marched away rather than cross the river and attack. Paulding wrote his mother that Gibbon claimed that "he had received orders from St. Paul to guard *this* side of the Yellowstone. There's literal obedience for you!"

Earlier, Paulding had begged to accompany a scouting party up the Bighorn River. Gibbon refused to let the doctor go. "I suppose he thinks," Gibbon wrote, "that any trifling assistance I might render toward smoothing over or preventing the death of half a dozen common soldiers or junior officers would not justify my absence in case of the commanding general being seized with a sudden attack of wind on the stomach."

George Custer, the impetuous field commander of the 7th Cavalry portion of Terry's column, made up for Gibbon's reluctance to fight. He disregarded orders to wait for Gibbon, and he led his exhausted men on a seventy-five-mile march with only five hours rest. Paulding, of course, did not know that at the time.

On the night of June 24, Gibbon's column camped on Tulloch's Fork, over twenty miles from the rendezvous where he was to meet Custer on the 26th. The next day, they broke camp early and marched over a high divide in the direction of the rendezvous at the mouth of the Little Bighorn on the Bighorn River. The infantry suffered so much from thirst that Paulding insisted they strike straight west for the Bighorn, downstream from the rendezvous point. After the leaders reached the river, Paulding said they needed three hours rest before moving on. He spent much of his time carrying water back to the exhausted soldiers who straggled behind.

After Gibbon's infantry made its camp, scouts reported seeing heavy smoke about thirty-five miles south.

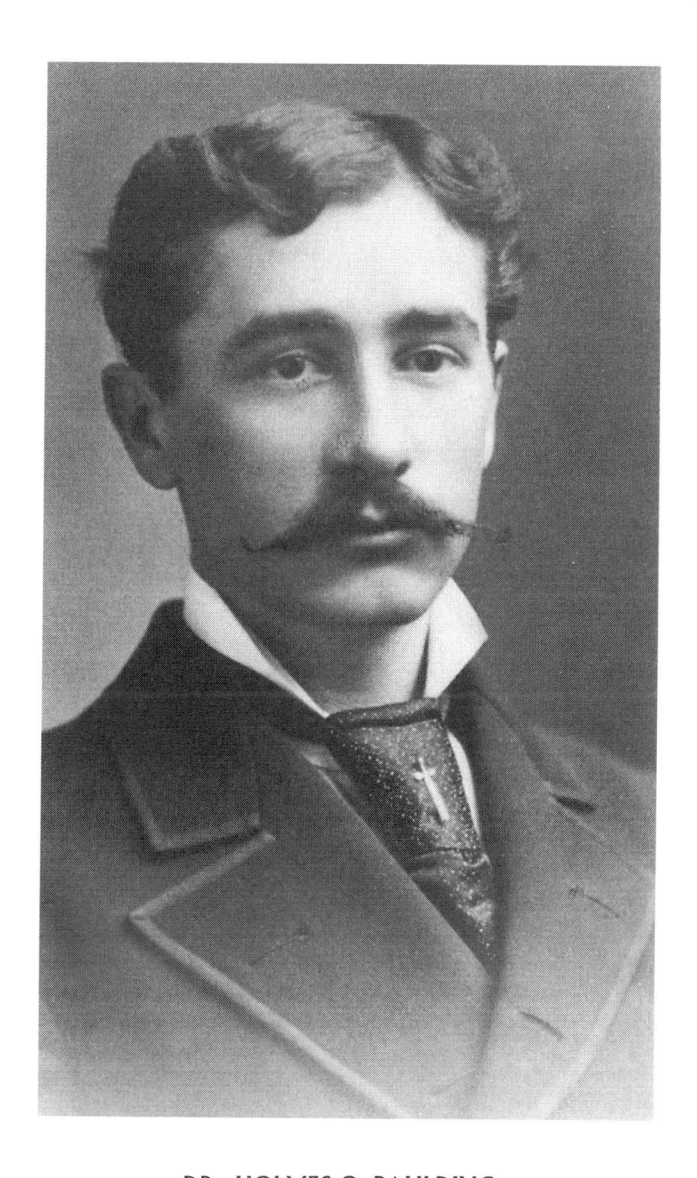

DR. HOLMES O. PAULDING

U. S. National Library of Medicine

None of Gibbon's delay had any effect on the battle. The same day that Gibbon's soldiers struggled over the divide from Tulloch's Fork to reach water—a march that General Terry said was one of the harshest tests ever faced by American soldiers—Custer attacked without waiting for the rendezvous. Gibbon's men thought the smoke they saw came from Custer burning what was left of the Indian Village. Actually it was the Indians burning timber to smoke out survivors of the battle.

While Paulding stayed back with the infantry, Gibbon's cavalry rode on ahead for twelve miles and camped some time after midnight. Looking after the exhausted soldiers kept Paulding up later. He might have got a little sleep before the infantry resumed its march at two, catching up with the cavalry at nine o'clock on the morning of June 26.

When they reached the cavalry, the infantry learned that three Indian scouts who had been with Custer had tried to get into the cavalry's camp. Thinking the scouts were hostile, Gibbon's cavalry repulsed them. The scouts had shouted over the river that Custer's personal command of five companies had all been killed. They said he had attacked a village of 1900 lodges and over 8000 warriors.

No one believed them. Paulding wrote that no one thought Indians could defeat such a gallant regiment. They concluded that Custer had tried to surprise a village of about two hundred lodges, thinking the surprise warranted an attack before the rendezvous with Gibbon's column.

Paulding wrote: "We expected to find a guard left behind with my dear old friend, Dr. Lord, in charge of the wounded, and I pictured to myself how glad he would be to have us come in and help him through. Custer, we supposed, would be scattered over the country pursuing fugitives."

They marched on, nearly twenty-six miles for the day, and two men were sent ahead to try and find Custer. At the same, a cavalry company was dispatched to explore the bluffs above the river. Paulding got permission to ride with them. They saw Indians ahead, and thought they were Custer's Arikara scouts. They rode forward to communicate, and the Indians opened fire. The company wanted to attack, but Gibbon ordered them back to camp. By then they realized the fire was burning timber, not an Indian village.

The next morning, June 27, Gibbon's column moved forward and found what was left of a hastily-departed Indian village. It had been two or three miles wide, and extended eight miles up the valley. They found Indian and cavalry saddles, cut-up blue clothing, and wounded cavalry horses. Two lodges left standing were filled with sixteen dead Indians. Others had been buried underground and on scaffolds, their horses sacrificed beside them. Bodies of white men were found, and also heads that had been cut off and dragged around by thongs. Paulding found a buckskin jacket worn by Lt.

James Porter of I Company, and the underclothing of Lieutenant Sturgis, an infantry officer riding with the Cavalry.

They found no signs of a battle within the village, but a lieutenant, scouting again to the bluffs, sent down a message that he had found two hundred dead bodies of white men. Now they knew the Indian scouts had told the truth. Later they met officers of the 7th Cavalry and learned the particulars of Reno's attack at the upper end of the valley. His battalion and Benteen's had, until the night before, been surrounded by three thousand Indians, a siege in which they sustained heavy losses.

Paulding was a personal friend of many of the 7th Cavalry officers from previous service at Fort Lincoln. Two of the three doctors assigned to the regiment had been killed. Paulding's old friend, army doctor George Lord, was killed with Custer; civilian doctor James De Wolf was killed with Reno. Both doctors were killed one day short of an important first year anniversary — Lord's promotion to first lieutenant and De Wolf's graduation from Harvard Medical School. Civilian doctor Henry Porter survived. He had cared for over fifty wounded before Paulding got there.

Paulding helped carry the wounded to the steamer *Far West* for transport down the Yellowstone and Missouri Rivers to Fort Lincoln. They shot seriously-wounded horses, skinned their hides into rawhide thongs, and used the rawhide to make litters, each carried by two mules, one in front and one behind. Three days and nights of evacuating the wounded, following immediately after the march over from Tulloch's Fork, exhausted Paulding.

In his July 15th letter to his mother, Paulding set out his ideas on how he thought hostile Indians should be handled:

"If we would only just quit issuing munitions of war, take possession of the agencies and burn them, take the families left by the warriors and remove them to a safe place as hostages, and hang every white man found selling arms and ammunition, it would settle the question in a month or two without bloodshed. . . . This sort of thing is liable to either toughen one tremendously or knock him up. It has had the effect of toughening me so that I never felt better in my life."

Nevertheless, the faithful doctor never learned to pace himself when soldiers needed medical attention. On April 21, 1883, while attending to his duties at Fort Sidney, Nebraska, he had heart failure. He died a week later, aged thirty-eight. The *Army and Navy Gazette* remembered him as "an able, accomplished, modest, faithful, hard-working officer, whose death involves a public loss."

Suggested reading: Thomas R. Buecker (Ed.), "A Surgeon at the Little Big Horn," in *Montana, The Magazine of Western History, v. 32, No. 4* (August, 1982).

DOCTOR GRANDMA

Emma French's first experience as a midwife came in 1856 when she marched with the Edward Martin handcart company of Mormons, bound for Utah. She cared for Mrs. Paul Gourley during childbirth in the freezing cold of Wyoming. Then she carried the new baby, Paul, across icy rivers to keep him dry. Almost a third of the company perished. Many of the others had amputations after reaching their destination. Gentle, tender-hearted Emma survived without permanent injury.

Emma had been raised in a destitute family in England, and she agreed to work for a year in Utah to pay for her transportation.

Emma married John D. Lee in January 1858. Reputedly he married over nineteen women. Emma bore him seven children. We don't know how many times he was present when Emma had his baby—he had so many wives to think about and much of the time he was on the dodge to avoid arrest for his role in the Mountain Meadows Massacre which occurred three months before Emma met him—but he certainly missed the last time Emma had his baby. For the birth of Victoria—named for the Queen of England—Emma relied on her 13-year-old son to help.

Lee fled to Arizona with Emma and perhaps another wife or two. He established a ferry across the Colorado River at the place still called Lee's Ferry.

Emma married Frank French in 1879 after Lee was executed. Frank, a tall, heavily built Civil War veteran, had come to Arizona in 1872 from California after his wife died. After ranching a few years and operating a hotel and boarding house in Holbrook, Emma and Frank moved to Winslow in May, 1887. Then Emma began caring for expectant mothers in what the family soon called the Baby Farm. With her experience in midwifery, both giving and receiving, it is not strange that Emma took up that work to help support the combined families. Emma, fifty-one years old, was five feet, four inches tall and heavy set with a determined set to her jaw. She set up a large room for her patients with two beds and a spare roll-away in a closet.

Emma insisted that cowboys, ranchers, and expectant fathers of all kinds give her notice at least three months in advance so she would have time to make the arrangements. The mother could stay as long in the Baby Farm after delivery as she wished.

Railroad men who could not bring their wives in were expected to keep Emma carefully posted as the due date approached. She required them to have other help in the home so she could return within a few hours after the child was born, assuming no complications. Sometimes an engine drawing a single railroad car would take Emma out and return for her after the ordeal was over.

In 1888, a year after moving to Winslow, Emma experienced the greatest sorrow of her life when fourteen-year-old Vicky, the baby born with the help of her brother, killed herself by drinking laudanum. The newspapers said the "vivacious, hearty girl had earlier that evening attended a dance in the highest spirits" and her death was "mysterious and unaccountable."

But this teen-aged girl had been rejected and reviled by other girls as well as boys after her father took all the blame for one of the most horrible tragedies in Old West history. The revulsion would continue to the fourth generation of John Lee's descendants. Vicky had been the prettiest, the most pampered and loved of Emma's children. Emma's sorrow at her death would never end.

Another family sorrow came four years later when Ike, the first of Emma's sons to marry, was shot and killed in his home. Ike's killer was a man named Wagner who had seduced Ike's wife. The cast in this all-too-common frontier scene with its twisted result included fourteen-month-old Victoria French, named after her father's favorite sister.

At first there was much talk of lynching Wagner. Then the women of the town said that if the men hanged Wagner, they would hang Ike's wife. This bizarre attempt at gender equality ended when the police hid Wagner from the male vigilantes, and the female variety of the species gave up the threat to turn an innocent baby into an orphan.

The people called Emma Doctor French and employed her in other cases of sickness and accident. She treated fevers, boils, injuries, and infections of all kinds.

When Emma left England her brother Henry was a well-known pugilist, middle-weight champion of the part of England where he lived. In the 1890s Henry wrote Emma that their parents had died and he was lonely and in bad health. Emma sent the money so Henry and a niece, as nurse, could come to Arizona. Emma was shocked at the broken old man who arrived, but she took both visitors into her family, gave the brother a private room, and cared for him until he died.

Stories began circulating in the community about Emma's healing power. In all her years as a midwife she never lost a mother, although a few babies were stillborn. She could heal sore eyes, carbuncles, and boils. The small case she carried seemed full of miracle remedies, and she knew how to use them all. One instance that became part of Arizona folklore happened in 1892 when two men in a drunken brawl seemed to be mortally wounded. One was shot in the lungs; the other cut to pieces with a knife. The sheriff decided to hold both men until the first one died so he could charge the other with murder. The only "physician" available had to be sobered up so he could examine the victims.

"No use to trouble about them," the doctor said. "They'll both be dead in a couple hours."

Someone shouted, "Go get Doctor French."

Emma had the men taken to the hospital where she probed for and removed the bullet in one and spent two hours sewing up the knife wounds of the other. Within two weeks both men were back in the saloon, buying drinks for each other.

Emma was always popular with her many grandchildren, both from the French side and from the Lee side. They called her Doctor Grandma and loved to have her visit. She knew many songs and riddles and games, and always carried little surprises. Her stories were legendary and inexhaustible. Schoolteachers often invited her to speak to their classes.

Perhaps Emma worked too hard, caring so long for so many people. She died in 1897, aged sixty-one. Frank had been gone from home for six months with his construction work. Emma had dreams about him, including a premonition that something tragic was about to happen. So she sent word that she would be glad to have Frank come home to see her.

Frank came, and she was overjoyed. They visited for an hour and then she said she would cook his favorite dish. She got up and started for the kitchen. She stumbled and sank to the floor, crying out, "Oh, Frank."

It seemed that the whole town of Winslow gathered outside her home. Women wept, wrung their hands, and moaned. Indian women stood in silent groups. Even prostitutes came. Everyone had a memory of kind hands that massaged away pain, of an understanding heart that accepted all persons and always held out hope and comfort; hope in this life and comfort about the life to come.

None of them knew about the young woman pulling a handcart through the snow with a sick woman in it, of carrying a teen aged boy across an icy stream on her back so his feet would not freeze, of sharing her own rations until she had lost half her weight. They did not know about operating a ferry on a dangerous river that would frighten many men, of being alone for weeks on end with only her small children to help with the chores.

They did know about her constant care for an irascible and unhealthy older brother, slowly dying in a foreign land. And, of course, each one knew from his or her own experience or from reports of friends about her years in Winslow. To them she was Doctor Grandma French, with healing in her hands and love in her heart.

The railroad crews took their trains through Winslow quietly, without bell or whistle, until after Emma's funeral.

Suggested reading: Juanita Brooks, *Emma Lee* (Logan: Utah State University Press, 1975).

FRONTIER NEUROSURGERY

ON March 1, 1883, a horse kicked Sergeant James Patterson of the 3rd United States Cavalry in the head. The native of Lancaster, Pennsylvania, was stationed at Whipple Barracks, near Prescott, the capital of Arizona Territory. Fellow soldiers took him to the post hospital, where he was examined and treated. The diagnosis was "Lacerated wound of the scalp."

A simple dressing had been applied, but the soldier didn't get any better. Thirty days later, the diagnosis was changed to "Compound fracture of the skull." Assistant Surgeon George McCreery, the army doctor in charge of the hospital, trephined the patient on April 9. The opening into the skull to relieve pressure on the brain measured a little more than an inch by an inch and a half.

McCreery was a well-trained doctor, as were most army doctors at that time. He had graduated from St. John's College in New York (now Fordham University) in 1874, and from Bellevue Hospital Medical School in 1877. Appointed an army doctor in 1880, he relieved Walter Reed as post surgeon at Fort Apache, and two years later was transferred to Fort Whipple.

We don't know why the initial examination missed the fracture in Patterson's skull, or if Doctor McCreery actually felt it with his fingers a month later. We do know that X-rays weren't discovered until twelve years later.

We don't know if the wound became infected, although McCreery's answers on his medical examination, a few years before, showed a thorough awareness of the importance of Lister's discoveries. These discoveries, made sixteen years before, established conclusively the need for antiseptic conditions in surgery.

We do know that Sergeant Patterson went into convulsions on May 31, and died the next day.

Doctor McCreery was on special duty with a scouting party when he learned of Patterson's death. He must have been surprised.

Suggested reading: John R. Green, M. D. "Neurosurgery on the Frontier" in *Montana, the Magazine of Western History, v. 7, no. 3* (July, 1967).

HOUSE CALLS IN A BIG HOUSE

The distinction of the family of Inshta Maza (Iron Eyes), last head chief of the Omahas, rivaled that of the Adams family in Massachusetts. Sometimes called Joseph La Flesche after his white father, the chief refused to have his daughters tattooed or his sons' ears pierced, although his standing in the tribe entitled them to that honor.

The chief often said, "I was always sure that my sons and daughters would live to see the time when they would have to mingle with the white people, and I determined that they should not have any mark put upon them that might be detrimental in their future surroundings."

Susan, the youngest child, contributed her part to the family's prestige. She became the first Indian woman to graduate from medical school. Her older brothers and sisters were born in tipis or earth lodges, but Susan was born in a frame house in 1868. She was not raised in the Omaha culture, but she never forgot her people. Their history, their wishes for the present, their hopes for the future were the beacons lighting her way through life.

Susan's oldest sister, a writer admired by Henry Wadsworth Longfellow, was the first woman to speak up for Indian rights. Her brother became a leading anthropologist.

Susan's father became a Christian and deeply regretted that he could not read the English bible. He wanted his children to be educated. He had the help of the Presbyterian missionaries on the Omaha reservation in Nebraska.

The missionaries thought it pointless to educate boys only to have them marry girls who expected to live in a tipi with a warrior. So they taught the girls domestic skills — care of the home, the animals, and the sick; preparation of food; the observance of the Sabbath. Fortunately for some, including Iron Eyes' family, academic training followed the vocational training.

When oldest sister Susette (Bright Eyes) finished the reservation school, she went to the Elizabeth Institute for Young Ladies in New Jersey. Younger sisters followed, and Susan was the last. After this school, seventeen-year-old Susan came back to the reservation and taught for two years at the reservation school.

During this employment Susan met Alice Fletcher, an anthropologist from Harvard and a fellow of Harvard's Peabody Museum. In fact, she treated Fletcher when Fletcher was ill from inflammatory rheumatism. Susan told the bedridden Fletcher that she would like to go to medical school.

"When I was little," she said, "I saw a woman die because the white

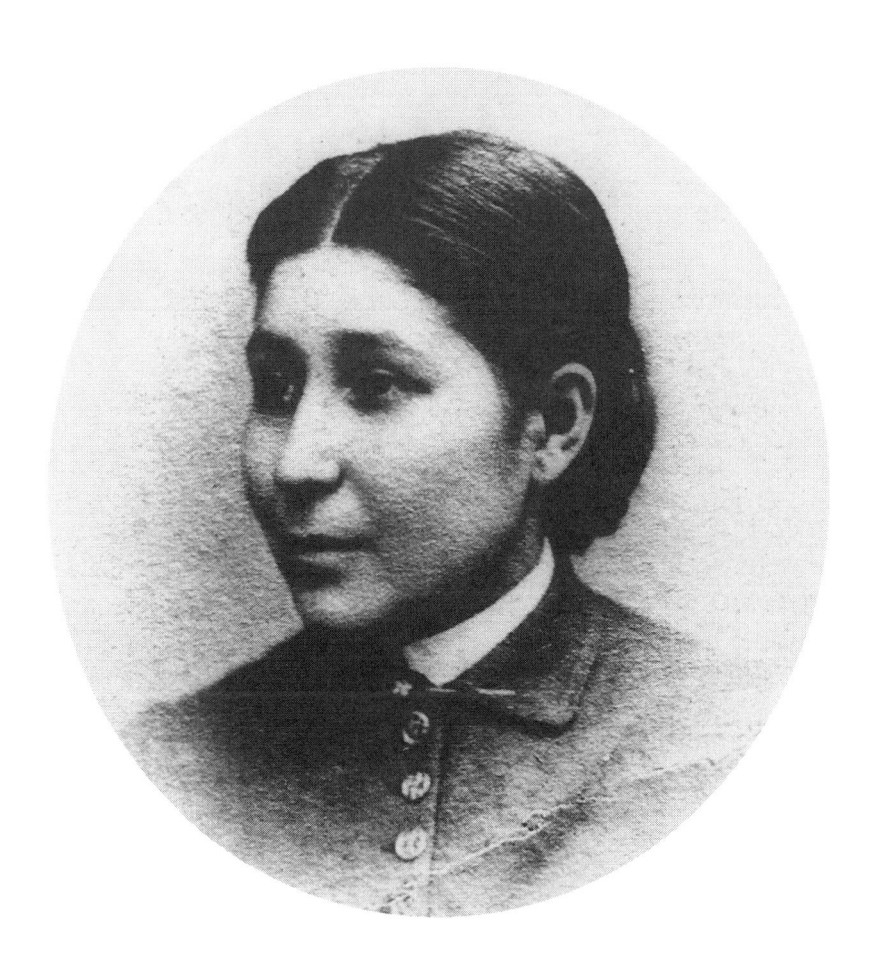

DR. SUSAN PICOTTE

National Anthropological Archives, Smithsonian Institution

doctor wouldn't treat her." Her face turned grave, and Fletcher listened quietly.

"I want to be a doctor," the young woman said.

"You'll have to go to college and make good grades, my dear."

"I can do that."

Susan went to the Hampton Institute in Virginia, one of the nation's finest colleges for non-white students. She graduated in 1886, second in her class. Her principal described her as a "young woman of unusual ability, integrity, and fixedness of purpose."

Dr. Martha Waldron, the resident doctor at the college, had graduated from the Woman's Medical College of Pennsylvania, and when she learned of Susan's burning desire to study medicine, she urged her to apply there. Alice Fletcher, who came to the graduation exercises, was delighted with Susan's record and also urged her to apply for medical school.

"Where will I get the money?" Susan asked.

"I'll see what I can do," Fletcher replied.

The anthropologist, who knew Susan and her family well, was able to secure scholarship funds from the United States Office of Indian Affairs, making Susan the first person in our nation's history to obtain federal aid for professional education. She also got assistance from the Women's National Indian Association.

Susan taught at Hampton during her first summer in medical school. She went home for the second summer, where she cooked, sewed, worked in the fields, harnessed horses, stacked hay, and even squeezed in some nursing during a measles epidemic.

Susan completed the three-year medical school, this time graduating first in her class. She interned a year in Philadelphia, and, in 1890, became the government physician for her Omaha tribe, responsible for over twelve hundred Omahas. She made house calls on foot or with a horse all over the thirty mile by forty-five mile reservation. In one month during 1891, she saw a hundred thirty patients.

Susan nursed her tribe through epidemics of influenza, cholera, and dysentery. She was never strong physically. The long walks and rides to call on her patients finally broke her health down. She had to resign from the tribal position in 1893. But she didn't forget her people.

The next year Susan married Henry Picotte, a mixed blood—French and Sioux—Indian. In the old days, the Sioux and the Omaha had been bitter enemies, but Susan said Henry was the "handsomest Indian she had ever seen." She and Henry settled in Bancroft, Nebraska, where Susan set up a private practice, serving both Indian and white patients. She became a leader in the state medical society and promoted health legislation in the state legislature.

Susan Picotte accepted the prevailing views of both Indians and whites about the place of women. She saw her medical practice as consistent with those views that a woman's place was in the home. Home was a sanctuary, a refuge for a tired husband at the end of the work day. There the woman was to rear children, instill moral values, and guard democracy. Susan went into those homes and taught her patients practical knowledge about cooking, cleaning, and nursing.

Susan said, "I feel that as a physician I can do a great deal more than as a mere teacher, for the home is the foundation of all things for the Indians, and my work I hope will be chiefly in the homes of my people."

Susan was an active prohibitionist, but her husband was a hard drinker. He died in 1905, leaving her with two small sons and an invalid mother needing care. Susan led a delegation to Washington in 1906 to lobby for the prohibition of alcohol on the reservation.

A lifelong problem with neurasthenia led to increasing deafness and constant back pain. Nevertheless, she continued to work as a physician, teacher, preacher (she was appointed by the missionaries), and field worker. She conducted church services in the Omaha language and held Christian burial services for the dead.

In 1913, three years before her death, Susan saw another lifelong dream come true, when she opened a hospital on the reservation at Walthill, Nebraska.

When Susan died in 1916, the local newspaper added an extra page to carry the eulogies. It said, "Hundreds of white people and Indians owe their lives to her treatment, care, and nursing. She rose to greatness and to great deeds out of conditions which seldom produce more than mediocre men and women, achieving great and beneficial ends over obstacles almost insurmountable."

This magnificent doctor for both Indians and whites was buried beside her husband in the Bancroft Cemetery.

Suggested reading: Valerie Mathes, "Dr. Susan La Flesche Picotte in L. G. Moses & Raymond Wilson, (eds.) *Indian Lives* (Albuquerque: University of New Mexico Press, 1985).

AGENCY DOCTOR

Both the father and grandfather of Thomas Bailey Marquis were physicians serving with the Union Army in the Civil War. Thomas, born in December, 1869, was the youngest of four children. Bright, although not studious, he graduated from school at seventeen. Thomas wanted to teach school, but he looked too young for anyone to hire.

Thomas loved to read about Indians, buffaloes, the plains, and the wild west. He worked as a printer on a newspaper in Saint Joseph, Missouri. When he was twenty-one, he went to Helena, Montana, to work on a newspaper there. He would never lose his fascination for Indians and the American West.

A year later, Thomas moved to a newspaper in Anaconda, where he met and married a local girl, Octavia Hillhouse. In 1894 he decided to become a doctor. Montana had no medical school, so he returned to Kansas City for his studies at the University Medical College. He graduated four years later near the top of his class. He returned to Anaconda in time to help Octavia deliver their first child, Minnie.

Doctor Marquis opened his first office in Ennis, Montana, with a bank loan to buy his office furniture. He soon had a green-broke horse for a fee, and he bought a buggy on credit from a traveling salesman. By the time Octavia and the baby joined him, he had the buggy paid for and the loan paid off. But Ennis and the Madison River Valley did not grow as he expected, so he moved to Bozeman for a few months and then on to Clyde Park in Park County.

The new doctor became a familiar figure in Park County as he made house calls to remote places. He enjoyed surgery in his beginning years. He thought most about relieving pain and suffering. He treated gunshot wounds, delivered babies by Caesarian section, and amputated many fingers and toes and some hands and feet. In later years he grew critical of unnecessary operations, and he realized that he was then saving hands and feet that he would have amputated earlier. He served as County Health Officer, and he spoke twice at conventions of the state medical association.

Thomas enjoyed music. He fashioned a wire holder to loop over his ears so he could play the harmonica and guitar simultaneously. The family worshiped in the Methodist church, where Octavia sang in the choir and Minnie played the organ. Younger daughter, Anna, had been born in Bozeman. They lost two other children in infancy.

Thomas' grandfather had been both an ordained minister and a physician. Thomas had the same intellectual curiosity and breadth. He read a friend's lawbooks until the friend suggested that Thomas take the state bar examination. He passed the examination in 1914.

The local Methodist minister, who had to supplement his church pay with day labor, sued an employer for unpaid wages. Thomas won the case for the minister. He declined further requests for legal services, saying he wanted to quit when he was one hundred percent successful.

By 1916 the Marquis marriage was on the rocks. Tomas joined the Army Medical Corps as a captain. He got to France just after the armistice. He was discharged in 1919 and returned to Montana, this time locating in Whitehall, Jefferson County.

Freed from marital responsibilities, he spent more and more time studying Indians and writing western history. In 1922 he became agency physician on the Northern Cheyenne Reservation at Lame Deer.

The doctor's understanding of and respect for the Indians soon overcame cultural barriers, and his patients became informers about a history, until then unrecognized. When he learned that several dozen survivors of the Little Bighorn Battle were still alive, Doctor Marquis embarked on the study and writing that would make him famous. By as late as 1930, seventeen Cheyennes who had been adult warriors in the Little Bighorn Battle were still alive.

But serving as physician for fourteen hundred Indians on a six hundred square mile reservation left little time to write. So he resigned his position in 1927 and opened a medical practice in Lodge Grass in the Crow Reservation, fifteen miles south of the battlefield that he would study for the remainder of his life.

After four years, he closed his medical practice completely and moved to nearby Hardin. There he established a small, private museum, to which he charged five cents admission.

Doctor Marquis learned sign talk, and he interviewed many survivors of the Custer battle, including Sioux, Cheyennes, Crows, and whites. He published five books and many articles, pamphlets, and stories about the battle. He purchased weapons and equipment used in the battle that had lain hidden in Indian lodges for a half century.

Marquis died of heart failure in 1935. As a veteran of World War One, he was buried with full military honors in the Custer Battlefield National Cemetery.

This doctor, lawyer, and writer had become a devoted friend and an accurate chronicler of Montana Indians.

Suggested reading: Thomas B. Marquis, *The Cheyennes of Montana* (Algonac, MI: Reference Publications, 1978).

DOCTOR SOFIE

In 1893 the residents of Brazoria, Texas—in the Brazos River bottomlands, fifteen miles above its mouth on the Gulf of Mexico—talked excitedly about the new doctor coming all the way from New York to settle there. Nearby Columbia had once been the capital of the Republic of Texas, and the Father of Texas, Stephen F. Austin, had died there while attending to government affairs. Brazoria had once been an important port and townsite in the Austin Colony, and many leaders in the independence movement had lived there. But now the economy was slow, medical doctors were more accepted on the frontier, and Brazoria needed one.

The citizens did not expect a forty-five-year-old widow who had fourteen grown children. Even the few who suspected that Sofie Herzog might be a woman probably expected a grandmotherly midwife, not a distinguished graduate of a Vienna, Austria, medical school who had trained with some of the best physicians in Europe. Doctor Herzog had managed a successful medical practice in New York City, and she moved to Texas for exactly the same reason that had motivated thousands of men during the previous seventy years — ADVENTURE!

Texas heat, short tempers, and the struggling economy produced gun battles, and the thick woods and bottomland marshes provided hideouts for outlaws. Natural enemies were alligators, water moccasins, malaria, and yellow fever. Brazoria needed a brave doctor, and Sofie fit right in.

At a time when fashionable women wore bustles and coiled their hair atop their heads, Sofie rode astride in a specially-made divided skirt, her man's sombrero shoved down on her short curls as she traveled from one patient to another. She soon had a thriving medical practice.

Dr. Sofie quickly established a reputation for removing bullets. She saved them, threaded them on a necklace, and wore the necklace proudly. She said it brought her luck, but her patients were the lucky ones.

Sofie's father had been a surgeon with an international reputation. When she was fourteen she married another surgeon. During their twenty-six years of marriage, they had fourteen children, four of them sets of twins. Sofie studied medicine as a way to help her husband, and she continued when he moved his practice to New York in 1886.

A few years later the husband died, and Sofie kept up the practice until 1893. Then she decided to follow her youngest daughter, Elfrieda Marie, and the daughter's husband, Randolph Prell, to Texas. She lived with them for a time and practiced out of the Prell house. Soon she had built a three room office with living quarters in rhe back. Prell worried about her living alone and offered her a gun, but Sofie didn't want it.

Even without a gun, Sofie could take care of herself. Once, when a visitor refused to leave her office, she chased him out with a fireplace poker.

Medicine on the frontier was not for the fainthearted. Essential implements were a saw for amputations and strong pliers for pulling teeth. Doctors had no antibiotics, and the main pain killer was whiskey. Bloodletting was a common therapy; Sofie could have got her leeches close at hand. Doctors relied heavily on quinine, mustard plaster, castor oil, and their own common sense.

In 1905 Sofie applied for the position of railway surgeon on the St. Louis, Brownsville, and Mexico railroad, then building into south Texas. She had already treated many of the railroad workers, and their praise got her the job. When the officials learned that they had hired a woman, they asked her to resign. She refused, saying she wouldn't leave as long as the patients were satisfied. For the next twenty years Sofie rode horseback, and on railroad cars, engines, and handcars to reach satisfied patients along the railroad line.

While she was tough, Dr. Sofie never forgot that she was a woman. She remained close to all of her children and loved to talk about her grandchildren. She kept a work basket of needlework in her office so she could sew or crochet when she had the time.

Sofie decorated her office with wild animal skins, mounted animal specimens, a collection of walking sticks, and her own medical museum. The museum contained several specimens of premature or still-born babies preserved in formaldehyde. One had two heads and three arms. A granddaughter had the babies buried when Sofie died. The other specimens went to the University of Texas Medical School.

The drier bottomlands had many rattlesnakes, and Sofie had many rattler skins in her collection. She would skin them herself and mount them for display on her walls. Once she said she would like to have an alligator, and one was promptly delivered. She thought it was dead; it was only stunned. When it began thrashing about in her office, she defended herself with the same fireplace poker she had used earlier.

Always ahead of her time, Sofie was one of the first in Brazoria with an automobile. She took driving lessons and soon made her rounds in a Ford runabout.

At sixty-five Sofie married Colonel Marian Huntington, five years older than she. She continued to practice medicine until she died in 1925. At her request, she was buried with the good luck necklace. It had twenty-four bullet slugs in it.

Suggested reading: Cindi Myers, "Daring Dr. Sofie," in *True West, v. 41, no. 7* (July, 1994).

DOC SUSIE

When Susan Anderson graduated from the University of Michigan Medical School in 1897, she was sure she had tuberculosis. She decided to establish a medical practice at her Cripple Creek, Colorado, home, hoping the dry air would improve her own health.

Four years later, after being jilted at the altar, she moved to Greeley. She worked there for six years as a nurse, often taking orders from doctors who knew less than she.

Susan's health had improved, but the tiredness returned at Greeley, and she knew the tuberculosis was active again. She decided to move on to the driest, coldest, most lonesome place she knew, hoping to either die or get well.

Fraser, Colorado, a lumbering town 8500 hundred feet high on the west side of the continental divide, had only one doctor. He worked for the railroad, but Susan hoped that some of the Swedish lumbermen would prefer a different doctor, even if the doctor was a woman. She moved into a tiny shack and took part-time work as a store clerk to pay the bills.

The first to call professionally was a cowboy.

"Ma'am," the shy cowboy began. "Dave got cut up real bad and he's all I got. Can you come, please?"

"Where is your friend?"

"Down at the corral."

"Well, can't you bring him here?"

"He ain't just my friend ma'am, he's my horse."

Susan was not surprised that her first house call was a horse call. In those days, doctors were also expected to treat animals and even pull teeth when no dentist was available. The horse recovered, and men began talking about the new doctor in town. She asked them to call her Doc Susie. She knew they would not call her doctor, and she wanted something more than a polite "ma'am."

Susan's health improved as her practice grew. The Swedish lumbermen began to accept her. One summer morning a young logger rode up and jumped from his horse.

"Doc Susie," he shouted. "You've got to come right now. Elof Nielsen broke his arm up St. Louis Crick, and the bones are sticking right out. They're bringing him down to Lapland. You got to come right now!"

The injured logger lay in a tent when Susan reached the lumber camp. She could see the bone ends protruding from the torn flesh.

"Do you know who I am?" she asked. She had not seen this one before.

"Ya, Doc Susie. I'm chur glad you come. Tree, she fall over, da wrong way."

Susan told the foreman to have the cook shack women start boiling water and to fix her some coffee. "I'll need you, Axel, and about three other strong men right here."

"Dey do dot already. Vater boilink okay. Efferbody know Doc Susie vant lotsa hot vater."

"You and three men, Axel — I need strong ones — you must take off your shirts and wash real good."

Axel Bergstrom selected the men. They frowned at each other as they took off their shirts and washed their arms.

"Clear to the armpits," ordered Susan. "I can fix the broken arm, but the greatest danger is from germs. We must keep germs out of the wound."

The men muttered, but they washed as she ordered. Then Susan explained how the helpers were to hold the injured man and what they were to do when she said, "pull, relax, twist left, twist right."

Susan removed Elof's bloody shirt and irrigated the wound with hot water, carefully picking away the dirt, bark, and lint.

When the four men took Elof's arm as she instructed, Susan poured ether on a pad and held it under Elof's nose. Then she barked commands to her helpers and the bones were soon properly aligned. She sewed up the wound and made a splint from cardboard boxes and shims from the tool shed. Elof said something in Swedish to Axel.

"He says ven are you cuttink his arm off?" Axel said.

Susan laughed and told Elof he would soon be back in the woods as good as new. She ordered a boy to kill all the flies in the tent and stay there to see that no more came in. She said she would stay in the camp overnight in case she was needed. The lumberjacks filed past, each one saying quietly, "tank you missus."

Susan Anderson never married. She retired in 1956, when she was eighty-six. She still loved the lumbermen, and they all loved her. She refused the offer of Ethel Barrymore to play her life on the stage. She died when she was ninety, a legend in Colorado.

Suggested reading: Virginia Cornell, *Doc Susie* (Carpinteria, California: Manifest Publications, 1991).

SWAT THE FLY

Samuel Crumbine was born in a log house in Pennsylvania in 1862. His blacksmith father died in a Confederate prison in the Civil War. After living most of his first eight years with a grandmother, Sam was placed in a soldiers' orphan school in Mercer, Pennsylvania.

At sixteen, Sam found work for board and room in a store owned by a pharmacist-physician. When he graduated from Cincinnati College of Medicine, he moved to Dodge City, Kansas, to practice. Besides treating patients in one of the wildest towns on the frontier, Sam—barely five feet six with a quick smile and bright, happy eyes—got interested in public health.

His initial work was improving the quality of drinking water. Then he started his most famous crusade, directed against the common housefly. Sam wanted to educate the public and show them how to rid their houses of flies. It was uphill work. People considered flies a nuisance, but they never bothered to do anything about them. Sam traveled over the state, lecturing on the danger, talking to newspapers, and meeting with other doctors. He published a "Fly Bulletin" and got the Boy Scouts interested in the project.

But nothing much was accomplished until sometime in the 1890s, when Sam took time off to attend a baseball game in Topeka. In the bottom of the ninth the score was tied at two. With one out and a Topeka runner on third, the fans started yelling as the next batter approached the plate.

"Sacrifice fly, sacrifice fly, sacrifice fly," the excited fans shouted. But the batter missed the first pitch.

Then a loud voice boomed out, "Swat the ball." Another fan near Sam repeated the call to swat the ball. Other fans joined in and Sam begin thinking: "Sacrifice fly . . . swat the ball . . . sacrifice fly . . . swat the ball." Then he said, almost to himself, "I have it, I have it: *Swat the Fly.*"

Sam was so excited he didn't see the next play, and he didn't tell us how the game came out. But he came out of the ball park with a slogan that would sweep the country and become part of our vocabulary.

The next Fly Bulletin had SWAT THE FLY in large capitals on the first page. Newspapers took it up, and the slogan spread. A teacher in Weir City wrote that he had cut a roll of wire screening into squares and tacked them to handles. Boy scouts had left two of the "fly swatters" in every home in town. Delighted, Sam passed the information on to a scoutmaster in Olathe, and his troop helped spread the clean-up movement.

Doctor Crumbine had a lifetime career in public health and achieved world-wide fame in the field.

Suggested reading: Samuel J. Crumbine, M D, *Frontier Doctor* (Philadelphia: Dorrance & Co., 1948.)

BESSIE AND THE BRONCO

The bank crisis of 1907 hurt Doctor Bessie Lee, practicing in Moville, Iowa. She was struggling to raise three orphaned nieces, and a fifth doctor, backed by a wealthy family and influential friends, had just moved to the town. Her father had practiced in South Dakota, and her brother was a doctor in Washington State. Bessie decided to move west.

It wasn't a spur-of-the-moment decision. Large areas of government lands, including Laramie County in Wyoming's southeastern corner, had been opened for homesteading. Promoters of settlement, including railroads, advertised special offers to persuade doctors, preachers, and teachers to emigrate, hoping that would improve the social climate and others would be encouraged to follow. The Burlington Railroad persuaded Bessie to homestead on land adjoining the proposed townsite of Carpenter, to be located thirty miles southeast of Cheyenne. She went out in July, filed on the homestead, and arranged to have a small house built.

When Bessie returned in December with her three young nieces, her house was the only permanent structure in Carpenter. A family building a a livery barn used its haymow for their own living quarters.

The train stopped two miles away at a ranch because Carpenter had no place to unload passengers. Her moving expenses and building the house left Bessie with seventy-five cents to her name.

The day after she arrived, a man came to say his horse was sick. The described symptoms indicated the animal had colic. Bessie mixed medicine four times as potent as she would give a human, and charged seventy-five cents. She not only doubled her treasury, but she gained an ardent supporter. After his horse recovered, he kept telling other settlers about the fine doctor who cured his horse without even an examination.

Bessie was the only doctor between Cheyenne and the Nebraska state line. Her territory extended into Colorado as far as Sterling. Sometimes a patient needing extended care could be put up in the hotel in Carpenter, but usually Bessie had to use her own home as a hospital.

She set one of her three small rooms aside for examinations. The unfinished room above became a hospital, furnished with three cots. Bessie and her nieces used the remaining two rooms as a kitchen-living room and a bedroom.

One fall evening Bessie was called to a homestead some distance from her office. When she completed her treatment and instructions, she started home with her buggy. The sky was clear, and the star-filled sky gave the high plains a peaceful aspect. Well acquainted with the trail back to Carpenter,

Bessie had no misgivings about leaving at the late hour. But soon the stars clouded over, the wind came up, and snow began to fall. She urged her horses on, but the wind rose to seventy miles an hour, and a tornado of snow bombarded them. Bessie could no longer see, her hands were numb, and her face burned from the icy pellets of wind-driven snow. The horses slowed to a creeping walk, and Bessie loosened the reins, hoping their instincts would lead them back to their own barn.

After the longest night Bessie could remember, her whole body was numb and she felt drowsy. She sensed that the horses had slowed from fatigue and were barely moving. Immediately alarmed, she forced herself to whip the horses and swing her own arms and legs. After a time, everything again seemed to slow down, and she wondered what would happen to the nieces, left homeless in the world for a second time. She saw that the horses had stopped before a faint light, barely visible in the furious storm.

It took a great effort for Bessie to climb out of the buggy and rap on the window. The horses had returned to the homestead shack that she had left three hours before. Her patient's husband helped her into the house, and now he treated her. Hours passed before she felt thawed out and warm again. She was able to return to the frightened little girls the next day. Bessie had other long, dangerous drives in hail, rain, and snowstorms, but that one remained the most frightening.

Bessie's fee in a confinement case was usually twenty-five dollars, plus mileage. She often had to take farm produce in payment, and sometimes she did not get that. Occasionally she would be called to some outlying place unfamiliar to her. Then she would have to cross the isolated plains in a farm wagon with a man about whom she knew nothing. Sometimes she felt uneasy, but it was still a world where a woman's life and honor were almost held sacred, and nothing bad happened.

One fall night she heard a knock on her door after she had gone to bed. She dressed hurriedly and met "two grim-looking swarthy Mexicans." Unable to speak English, they handed her a note. It said the writer's wife was having labor pains in a small Colorado town, and the men would bring her down in a railroad handcar.

Bessie's questions were answered with shrugs, nervous smiles, and hand motions. She re-read the note, decided that a human life might be at stake, and decided to go. She grabbed her medicine and instrument bag and followed the men to the Burlington tracks, where a third man waited by a handcar. The men indicated where she was to sit, made her comfortable, and began pumping the car down the tracks. Bessie sat on the edge with her feet dangling over the side, looked up at the starry sky, and enjoyed the trip. When the car stopped, the men escorted her politely to a house, bowed deeply, smiled broadly, and disappeared into the night. The husband and his wife were thankful that Bessie beat the stork by a hour.

Bessie never had a nurse. Cheyenne had a small nursing school, but its graduates always found city employment. Bessie served as nurse, dietitian, and scrubwoman in her small, second-floor hospital. When she began her practice she carried her own stock of standard drugs. Sometimes she had to make special trips to Cheyenne for hot water bottles, crutches, and poultices. The nearest dentist was in Cheyenne, and sometimes her patients could not afford the trip. Then she pulled teeth.

She had no instruments to measure blood pressure and no way to take X-rays. She had to depend on the touch of her fingers to set broken bones. When she was called out in accident cases, she would usually do her work on the homesteader's kitchen table.

Bessie most dreaded the pneumonia bacillus. Once it got into the patient's lungs, it took its deadly toll. She had no modern drugs or oxygen tent. Often she felt that she could do nothing more than use old remedies, proven reliable from experience. She would make the patient as comfortable as possible, trusting the human body to fight its own battle. But listening to the desperate gasping for air while the family wrung their hands in helpless fear made Bessie think she was a knight sent out to fight an armored dragon with a rusty, broken sword.

When Bessie was a medical student she examined flies under a microscope and she never forgot the loads of filth they carried. When she attended a mother having a baby in a shack with no screens on the door or windows, with the family dogs and cats and pet lambs—one time a tame antelope—crowded together with no closets other than nails in the walls for hanging up soiled clothing, and when she saw flies taking baths in the milk pitcher or water pail, she felt queasy in her stomach. Bessie always sterilized her instruments before leaving her office, and she carried them wrapped in sterilized towels. She also carried her own sterilized sheets and linens.

In desperate cases she would sometimes seek help from the husband. But husbands were usually a hindrance in confinement cases. Clumsy and confused, they acted as though they were in labor rather than their wives. About all they could do was bring in water and keep the stove going.

One time, Bessie had been on duty day and night for two weeks without ever spending a whole night in a bed. She had to have some sleep before going on to the next patient. The family had only one bed, so she wrapped herself in her coat and lay on the floor in a kitchen corner. The family went on with their work, walking around their doctor as she slept.

In July, 1908, the first school between Hereford, Colorado, seven miles south, and Burns, Wyoming, thirteen miles north, opened. Seventeen pupils, including Bessie's nieces, attended. The Methodists and the Disciples of Christ, using two retired ministers who had homesteaded, alternated at worshiping in the schoolhouse. They had no musical instrument, so sometimes they had to stop midway through the first verse of a hymn and start over, having started too low or too high.

Young men in the community greatly outnumbered young women. One day while Bessie was in the grocery store she saw a forlorn young man, and she made it a point to speak to him. While they talked he mentioned that he liked to play chess but no one in Carpenter knew how.

"My father taught me to play," Bessie said, "and I enjoy the game."

When their conversation ended she mentioned that she would have to play him sometime and try to beat him. The very next evening he knocked at Bessie's door, looking awkward in his Sunday best. Thinking he was a patient, Bessie invited him in. After they played a game of chess, he seemed disappointed when she said she had work to do and gently moved him to the door.

Two days later he returned, holding up his injured hand and grinning widely. The sliver was so insignificant Bessie said there was no charge. It took her some time to ease him out the door that time.

He returned in two days with another splinter. This time Bessie removed it without saying a word, applied a dressing, and said in a cold, professional tone, "That will cost you a dollar."

The stunned young man understood what Bessie was telling him. He had no more splinter accidents, and Bessie lost her patient.

Bessie enjoyed life on the frontier. The only doctor between Cheyenne and Nebraska, she had developed a successful practice, her nieces were growing and beginning to help at home, and she enjoyed the freedom of western life, thinking she would never move. But a Wyoming bronco changed everything.

In summer, 1909, Bessie was called to Burns on an obstetrical case and had dinner in the town's small hotel. Surrounded by homesteaders, cowboys, ranchers, and the men who ran the livery stable, Bessie noticed a young man who looked different from the others. He was tall, the picture of health, and, as much as she could tell, his conversation was animated and his laughter contagious. She watched a while and asked the waitress who he was.

"Why, he's our student minister at the Lutheran church," the waitress replied.

Bessie, an active Methodist, had nothing serious against preachers, but from her youth she had thought they were not as virile and independent as other men. They seemed to lack some of the basic manly qualities. She remembered a conversation with friends as a young teen-ager about the kind of man they wanted to marry. She had said she would never marry a preacher.

But on the way back to Carpenter, she kept thinking about the young preacher at the other table. She didn't know why. She met new people almost every day, and none had ever aroused her curiosity like this.

About three o'clock the next morning a knock sounded at her door. It was the liveryman from Burns with a new patient, the young preacher. The lower part of his trousers was shredded and soaked in blood. He hobbled in and explained that he had been visiting in his parish. When he rode back after dark, his horse hit a barbed wire fence, and in plunging free, gave his rider a deep gash to the bone.

It took Bessie two hours to clean the wound because the people in Burns had filled it with flour to stop the blood. She ligated several blood vessels, sutured a large muscle that had been severed, trimmed the ragged edges, and mended the surface tissues as best she could. She had no anesthetic. Throughout the procedure, the preacher watched the repairs with interest, asked intelligent questions, joked about women doctors, discussed questions of medicine, and talked about life in the West. The liveryman, overcome at the sight of blood, had to leave the room.

His name was Alfred Rehwinkel, he was a seminary student in St. Louis, and a few years younger than Bessie. She didn't think a Lutheran minister was allowed to marry outside the denomination, particularly to a woman who could not speak one of the Scandinavian languages. But she told him he had to keep his leg elevated, and he could not go back to Burns so soon. She would keep him on a cot in the treatment room and give him the care he needed. She sent the liveryman home and started breakfast. Alfred ate like a hungry cowboy at a roundup.

Bessie had to make a call after breakfast. When she returned, Alfred was reading a Shakespearian drama he had found in her library. The days and weeks that followed were among the most memorable in Bessie's life.

Alfred's seminary graduated him early so he could fill an urgent call to a circuit-riding parish in Alberta. The parish extended into eastern and central British Columbia. It took almost three years after the bronco accident before the problems were all worked out. The oldest niece went into nurse's training, the second into teacher training, and the youngest went with Bessie to Canada. Bessie dusted off her German texts from college, and studied them with a new interest.

She gave up medicine to become a preacher's wife in Canada. Bessie and Alfred had two daughters and a son. The son became a preacher, and one of the girls married one. To the end of her long life, Bessie had kindly thoughts about a Wyoming bronco.

Suggested reading: Alfred M. Rehwinkel, *Dr. Bessie* (Saint Louis: Concordia Publishing House, 1963.)

ORDERING INFORMATION

Our True Tales of the Old West
are projected for 38 volumes.

For Titles in Print,
Ask at your bookstore
or write:

PIONEER PRESS
P. O. Box 216
Carson City, NV 89702-0216
(775) 888-9867
FAX (775) 888-0908

Other titles in progress include:

Californios	Frontier Militiamen
Western Duelists	Ghosts & Mysteries of the Old West
Frontier Lumbermen	Visitors in the Old West
Old West Artists	Scientists & Engineers on the Frontier